ARTHRITIS
the eSSential
guide

WAYNE RUTTER, GP

P 12

P 14

P 35

DEDICATION

For Heather
Thanks Mum

Published by ABC Books for the
AUSTRALIAN BROADCASTING CORPORATION
GPO Box 9994 Sydney NSW 2001

Copyright © Wayne Rutter 2003

First published February 2003

National Library of Australia
Cataloguing-in-Publication entry
  Rutter, Wayne, 1959
  Includes index.
  ISBN 0 7333 1085 0.

  1. Arthritis – Handbooks, manuals, etc.
  2. Arthritis – Treatments – Handbooks, manuals, etc.
  I. Australian, Broadcasting Corporation.

616.722

Designed by Ingo Voss, Vossdesign
Illustrated by Edwina Riddell
Set in 10.5/14pt Caslon Book
Colour reproduction by Colorwize, Adelaide
Printed and bound in Australia by Griffin Press, Adelaide

5 4 3 2 1

CONTENTS

About the author

Wayne Rutter has been a GP for the past 12 years and is currently practising as a family doctor in north-western Tasmania. He has a particular interest in rheumatology. He is Senior Clinical Lecturer in General Practice at the University of Tasmania.

Acknowledgments

I want to thank the three men who taught me everything I know about rheumatology and arthritis. First of all, thanks to Dr John York, former head of the Rheumatology Department at the Rachel Forster Hospital and Royal Prince Alfred Hospital in Sydney, a grandfatherly figure who helped me when I was a blustering intern. Next, thanks to Dr James Croker, my registrar when I was an intern at the Rachel Forster and who is now a rheumatologist in Tamworth. He happily imparted his wisdom and taught me how to stick a needle into nearly every joint in the body. Finally, thanks to Dr Peter Youssef, now a rheumatologist at Royal Prince Alfred Hospital, my contemporary, whose amazing razor-like knowledge of medicine, and particularly rheumatology, has always astounded me. In fact, he is still teaching me.

I would also like to thank Rose Creswell and Annette Hughes at Camerons Management for their efforts in finding a publisher, and John Marsden for encouraging me to write. Also many thanks are due to the talented team at ABC Books who polished and produced the book.

And lastly - Carrie, David, James and Michael. Love you.

CHAPTER | I

WHAT IS ARTHRITIS?

Any joint in the body

What is a joint?

Inflammation

A rthritis—the scourge of old age. That's how most people think about arthritis. But the truth is arthritis also affects young and middle-aged people. And because our life expectancy is increasing, more and more people in Western society are getting arthritis. In Australia, arthritis affects over 3 million people or 16.5 per cent of the population.

Studies have shown that arthritis has an impact on work, income, leisure time, housing, transport needs and social support. People with arthritis have up to 15 times greater work disability than non-arthritic people and 25 per cent of people with arthritis have a lowered income. Arthritis gives you chronic pain and loss of mobility and function that can seriously affect your life. Not being able to go for a walk or play a round of golf when you're feeling otherwise healthy can be a frustrating experience. Even daily routine activities such as bathing, dressing and eating with a knife and fork may become difficult. Some forms of arthritis are relatively mild, but others can destroy the joints, sometimes even leading to being in a wheelchair. Yet, most people with arthritis lead reasonably normal lives. It's important to see your doctor when symptoms first begin so that a prompt diagnosis can be made and early treatment initiated. Try to get out and do what you want to do. If the activity is aggravating your pain, find another way of doing it or find something else that gives you enjoyment.

WITH A POSITIVE ATTITUDE, LATERAL THINKING AND GOOD MEDICAL TREATMENTS, THERE IS NO REASON WHY YOU CAN'T DO MOST THINGS IN LIFE, EVEN IF YOU HAVE ARTHRITIS.

ANY JOINT IN THE BODY

Arthritis can affect any joint in the body, from the large obvious joints, such as the knee or the hip, to the joints between the jaw and skull, and the joints between the tiny bones of the middle ears. The distribution of its attacks often shows what type of arthritis you have. Rheumatoid arthritis often affects the small joints of the hands and feet, osteoarthritis usually affects the larger joints, such as the knees and hips, and gout seems to like

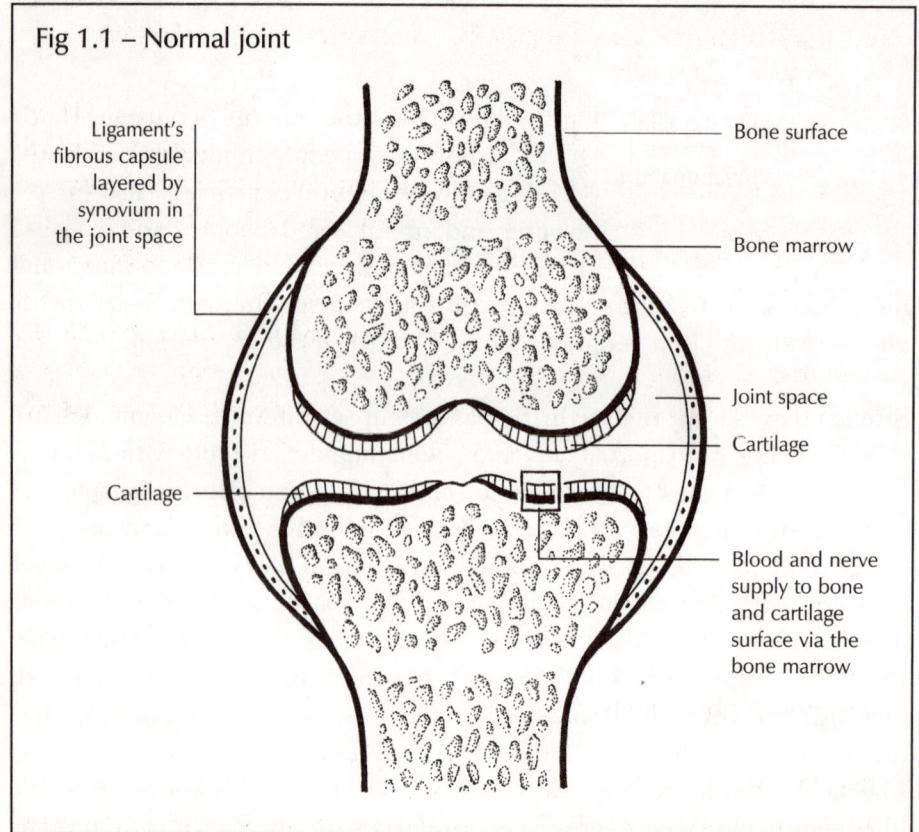

Fig 1.1 – Normal joint

Ligament's fibrous capsule layered by synovium in the joint space

Bone surface

Bone marrow

Joint space

Cartilage

Cartilage

Blood and nerve supply to bone and cartilage surface via the bone marrow attacking the joint between the big toe and foot. Joint stiffness—a common symptom of arthritis—can also help to show the type of arthritis. If you have an inflammatory condition, such as rheumatoid arthritis, you're likely to have stiff joints in the morning (lasting more than 30 minutes) that is especially noticeable when you get out of bed because prolonged rest actually aggravates joint stiffness. The stiffness can often last several hours and only improves with activity. On the other hand, if you have a non-inflammatory arthritis, such as osteoarthritis, joint stiffness (lasting less than 30 minutes) is aggravated by short periods of rest and improves with activity.

WHAT IS A JOINT?

A joint is a complex structure, with the sole function to provide flexibility of movement for the body (see Figure 1.1). Without that flexibility you'd feel like the Tin Man from *The Wizard of Oz*. There are different types of joint, such as the ball-and-socket joint of the shoulder and the hinge joint of the elbow.

The joint is made up of nine different types of tissue, all of which help maintain either the structure and function of the joint or the health of the joint.

Bones

Bones provide the architectural structure to the joint. They continually renew themselves, or 'remodel', a dynamic process in which two different types of bone cells act in equilibrium (see Figure 1.2). The first type of cells are *osteoblasts* which continually lay down the proteins collagen and glycoproteins. The proteins, which form the structure of a bone, are then mineralised and hardened by calcium. The second type of bone cells are *osteoclasts*. Their role is to scavenge old bone. When these two types of cells work in a regulated way, you have healthy bones. If they are out of synchronisation you will get bone problems, such as osteoporosis.

Cartilage

Cartilage acts as a cushion, or shock absorber, between the two bones of a joint. Cartilage cells, *chondrocytes,* produce jelly-like mucopolysaccharides and glycoproteins which, together with a small amount of collagen, form the substance of cartilage tissue. Cartilage is not mineralised with calcium and so doesn't become hard.

Synovial Membrane

Synovial membranes provide the clear, treacle-like fluid that lubricates the joint and makes its movements frictionless. The synovial membrane lines the inside of the joint capsule, tendon sheaths and bursae and is composed mostly of synovial cells.

Bursae

Bursae are sacs of synovial fluid that act as lubricating elements for the surrounding structures of the joint such as overlying muscles and tendons.

Joint Capsule

The joint capsule encloses the joint, providing integrity and helping the ligaments provide stability to the joint. The capsule is composed of a fibrous tissue, mostly collagen interspersed with fibrocyte cells (which produce the collagen).

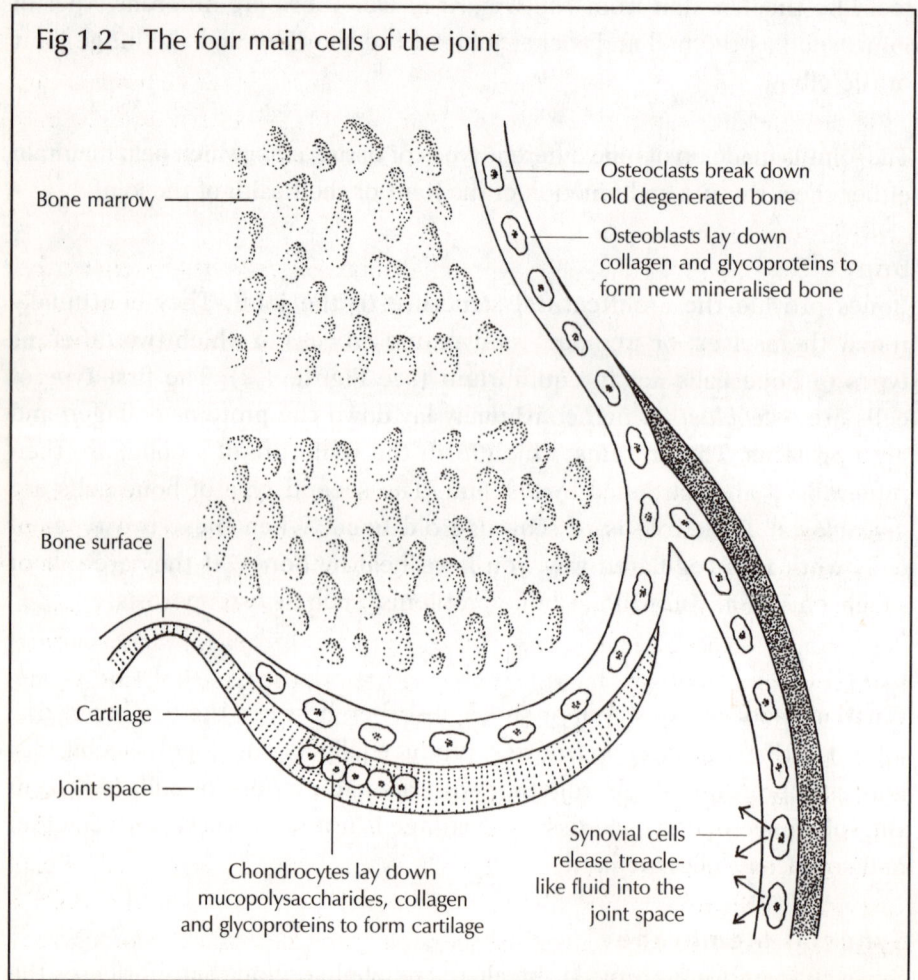

Fig 1.2 – The four main cells of the joint

Bone marrow

Osteoclasts break down old degenerated bone

Osteoblasts lay down collagen and glycoproteins to form new mineralised bone

Bone surface

Cartilage

Joint space

Chondrocytes lay down mucopolysaccharides, collagen and glycoproteins to form cartilage

Synovial cells release treacle-like fluid into the joint space

Ligaments

Ligaments are the main tissues providing stability to a joint. They are fibrous and consist mostly of collagen and fibrocyte cells. The fibres run generally in one direction, providing the bracing between the bones of the joint; for example, the knee joint has four ligaments—the anterior and posterior cruciate ligaments that give the knee front-to-back stability, and the medial and lateral collateral ligaments that give sideways stability.

Muscles and Tendons

Muscles are not actually part of a joint, but when the muscle fibres contract and shorten they provide the power of movement for a joint. The muscle is attached to a tendon, which is like the string of a pulley, and pulls on the bone to which it's attached, thereby giving joint movement.

Nerves

Nerves are essential to the function of a joint as they inform the brain about the joint's current position. The brain then controls the body's balance and posture. Without nerves, we would be completely uncoordinated.

Blood Vessels

Blood vessels provide the nutrients needed by joint cells; they remove the toxins that are produced in a joint with tissue breakdown and cell metabolism, and provide access to white blood cells needed for the repair and health of a joint.

INFLAMMATION

The literal meaning of the word 'arthritis' is joint (arthr) inflammation (itis). There are other types of inflammation associated with arthritis, such as tendonitis (inflammation of a tendon), synovitis (inflammation of the lubricating synovial layer around the joint) and capsulitis (inflammation of the fibrous capsule that surrounds a joint). All these surrounding structures of a joint can be inflamed at the same time as the joint. Some types of arthritis can even affect distant organs of the body at the same time. Lung, kidney, heart, brain, liver, muscle, eyes and skin can all be involved. Pain, heat and swelling are symptoms of inflammation — you get inflammation when your body's immune system tries to fix the cause of the arthritis. Unfortunately, when the body's repair system is activated, it can lead to debilitating symptoms. It's the same process when the body's immune system encounters an abscess or boil. The skin becomes red, angry and painful, and the local skin temperature increases.

THERE ARE OVER 170 DIFFERENT TYPES OF ARTHRITIS.

There are over 170 different types of arthritis, classified as inflammatory and non-inflammatory arthritis. Two of the most common are osteoarthritis and rheumatoid arthritis.

TYPES OF ARTHRITIS

INFLAMMATORY	NON-INFLAMMATORY
Rheumatoid	Traumatic
Systemic lupus erythematosus	Osteoarthritis
Scleroderma	Neuropathic (nerve damage)
Psoriasis	
Gout	
Sarcoidosis	
Sero-negative arthritis	
Juvenile arthritis	
Ankylosing spondylosis	
Dermatomyositis	
Reiter's syndrome	

OTHER FACTORS ASSOCIATED WITH INFLAMMATORY ARTHRITIS

Infections

Bowel disease

Vasculitis (blood vessel inflammation)

Amyloidosis

Cancers

Genetic diseases

Drug use – both medicinal and recreational

FACTORS ASSOCIATED WITH OTHER FORMS OF ARTHRITIS

Cancers

Congenital history

Response of the Immune System

When your body is attacked by a foreign body, the immune system responds by protecting itself. When a joint becomes inflamed, white blood cells (see Figure 1.3) kill the invading germs and help in the repair process. Although the immune system is wonderfully efficient in these processes, it sometimes doesn't know when to switch off, and that's when inflammatory arthritis takes a hold.

The immune system can tell the difference between a foreign germ and the body's cells because the germ cell contains proteins and other molecules that trigger the immune system. If the germ cell's proteins and molecules are the same or similar to the body's cell wall proteins and molecules, the immune system can't tell the difference between the germ cell and the body's cells. So the immune system clears the body of all germs, but because it identifies the body's cell as a germ, it attacks the body's cells too. If that particular germ has cell wall proteins and molecules similar to the joint cell, the immune system attacks the joint as well, resulting in an inflammatory arthritis. If the germ has cell wall proteins and molecules similar to, say, heart muscle cells, the immune system will also attack the heart, inducing cardiac myositis or cardiomyopathy. Some types of virus germs are particularly notorious for this.

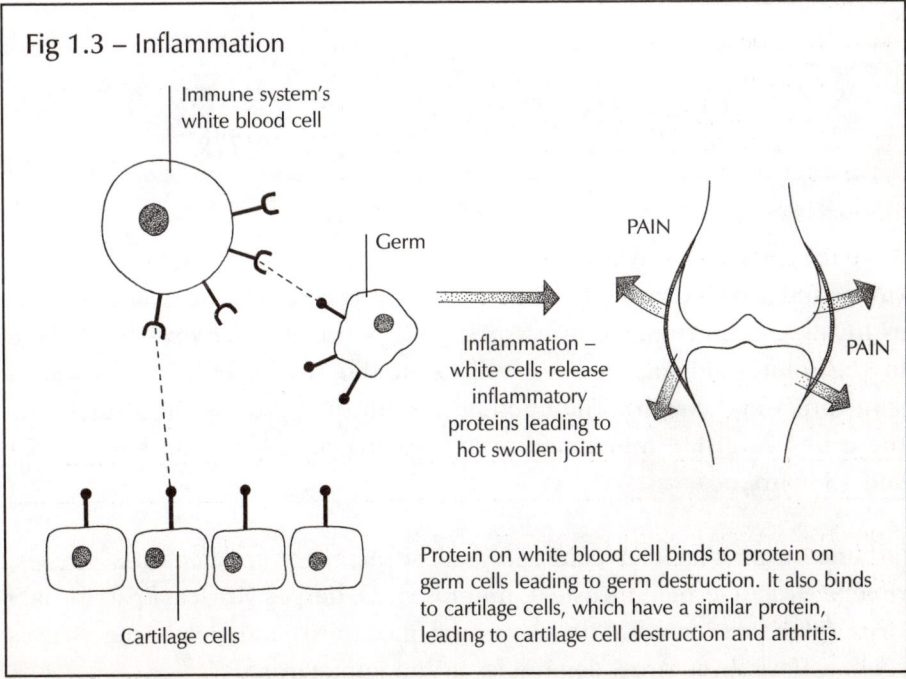

Fig 1.3 – Inflammation

Immune system's white blood cell

Germ

PAIN

Inflammation – white cells release inflammatory proteins leading to hot swollen joint

PAIN

Cartilage cells

Protein on white blood cell binds to protein on germ cells leading to germ destruction. It also binds to cartilage cells, which have a similar protein, leading to cartilage cell destruction and arthritis.

The similarity between germ cell molecules and human cell molecules explains why some types of arthritis are genetically influenced. There is not usually a direct inheritance of arthritis, but your genetic make-up determines the structure of your cells and influences whether or not you will develop arthritis. Even if you have the same cell structure as your affected parent, you'll still need to be exposed to a triggering factor for arthritis to start. Possible triggers for arthritis include environmental factors, such as chemicals; foods (and their colourings and preservatives); and allergens including house dust mite, pollens and grasses.

Viruses and other Germs

Fortunately, genetic differences between individuals are what gives the majority of us protection against the long-term inflammation of the body's organs. Only an unlucky small percentage of people are genetically made so that their cell wall proteins and molecules are similar to germ cell wall proteins and molecules, leading to the inflammation. The other problem for humans is that germs are continually mutating—it may be that a germ is not a problem, but it later mutates in a particular way, so that its cell wall proteins become similar to human cells. The ability of germs to mutate rapidly is why bacteria develop resistance to antibiotics and why the HIV/AIDS virus has managed to become infectious in humans when it was originally restricted to chimpanzees.

A VIRAL OR BACTERIAL INFECTION MAY
BE A TRIGGER FOR YOUR ARTHRITIS.

A typical cause of a short-term, single-joint arthritis is a virus. One common virus familiar to everyone is influenza. When you get the flu, you often feel as if you've been run over by a truck. This is because the virus has lodged in the joints and muscles (as well as in the throat and lung, giving a sore throat and cough). The immune system then attacks the virus inside these tissues giving inflammation and aching usually lasting between 24 and 48 hours.

Other viruses that can commonly cause arthritis are hepatitis viruses, rubella virus (German measles), mumps virus, herpes viruses, Epstein-Barr virus (glandular fever), HIV virus, and mosquito- and tick-borne viruses such as Ross River virus, dengue fever and hantavirus.

Bacteria

Bacteria are also known to cause arthritis, both directly and indirectly. In the direct mechanism, or septic arthritis, the bacteria is introduced into the joint by either a penetrating wound or surgery, or spread through the blood from an infection somewhere else in the body. The classic bacteria for blood-spread septic arthritis is *Neisseria gonorrhoeae*, which causes a sexually transmitted disease. The indirect mechanism for bacteria to cause arthritis is the same as for inflammatory arthritis—the immune system can't tell the difference between the bacteria and the body's cells. The immune system kills the bacteria but can't switch off because it continues to identify the body's cells as bacteria, so the inflammation continues. Some examples of bacteria bringing on these types of arthritis are Lyme disease caused by a spirochaete bacteria *Borrelia burgdorferi*, which is spread by ticks; rheumatic fever caused by *Streptococcus group A*; and scrub typhus, caused by *Orientia tsutsugamushi*, which is found in northern Australia, the Pacific Islands, South-east Asia, India, Central Asia and Russia.

Rheumatoid arthritis is thought by some to be initiated by the bacterial *mycoplasma*, which causes a lung pneumonia, although this view is not widely accepted by the medical community. Recent research shows rheumatoid arthritis may be caused by an infection with *parvovirus B19*, as 77 per cent of synovial tissue samples of rheumatoid patients in a study were positive for *parvovirus B19* DNA, and all were positive for a B19 protein called VP-1 compared with none for osteoarthritis. Synovial cells of rheumatoid patients were also able to spread *parvovirus B19* to uninfected cells in the laboratory. Parvovirus causes a childhood viral illness called slapped cheek syndrome, which produces bright red cheeks.

The discovery of which germ induces a particular form of arthritis will produce a major breakthrough in curing that arthritis. When we know the identity of the culprit, we can start immunising for that germ and so prevent further episodes.

CHAPTER | 2

TREATMENT OPTIONS

T here are some wonderful treatments for arthritis—both from the traditional medical fraternity and the not so traditional. There are also occasionally cases of quackery and misdiagnosis from both. Because I am medically trained I have a preference for medical treatments, although I believe complementary therapies can also be helpful. If you find something that helps, stick to it—medical and non-medical therapies can work well together.

Many of the medical therapies, if they are used appropriately and are monitored regularly, are safe to use long term. They can make a huge difference to your arthritis and vastly improve your lifestyle. You do need to find a doctor who's familiar with the drugs involved, as mistakes from using these drugs are most likely to happen because of a lack of familiarity. Specialist rheumatologists usually prescribe these drugs, and family doctors may have little experience with them. It's important for your family doctor to be aware of any possible side effects of medication so that follow-up monitoring tests can be made.

There are two main categories of drugs used in arthritis. The first group is used to improve symptoms only—the drugs have no effect on the disease activity. These drugs usually relieve symptoms within 60 minutes. Examples are paracetamol, codeine, prednisolone or cortisone, aspirin, naproxen and other associated non-steroidal anti-inflammatory medications. The second group of medications, or disease modifying drugs, switch off the inflammatory arthritis. They too provide symptom relief, but the onset is slow and can take up to three months to be effective. These drugs are potent and need meticulous follow-up by whoever has prescribed them. (See Figure 2.1.)

SOME DRUGS IMPROVE SYMPTOMS ONLY;
OTHERS SWITCH OFF THE INFLAMMATION.

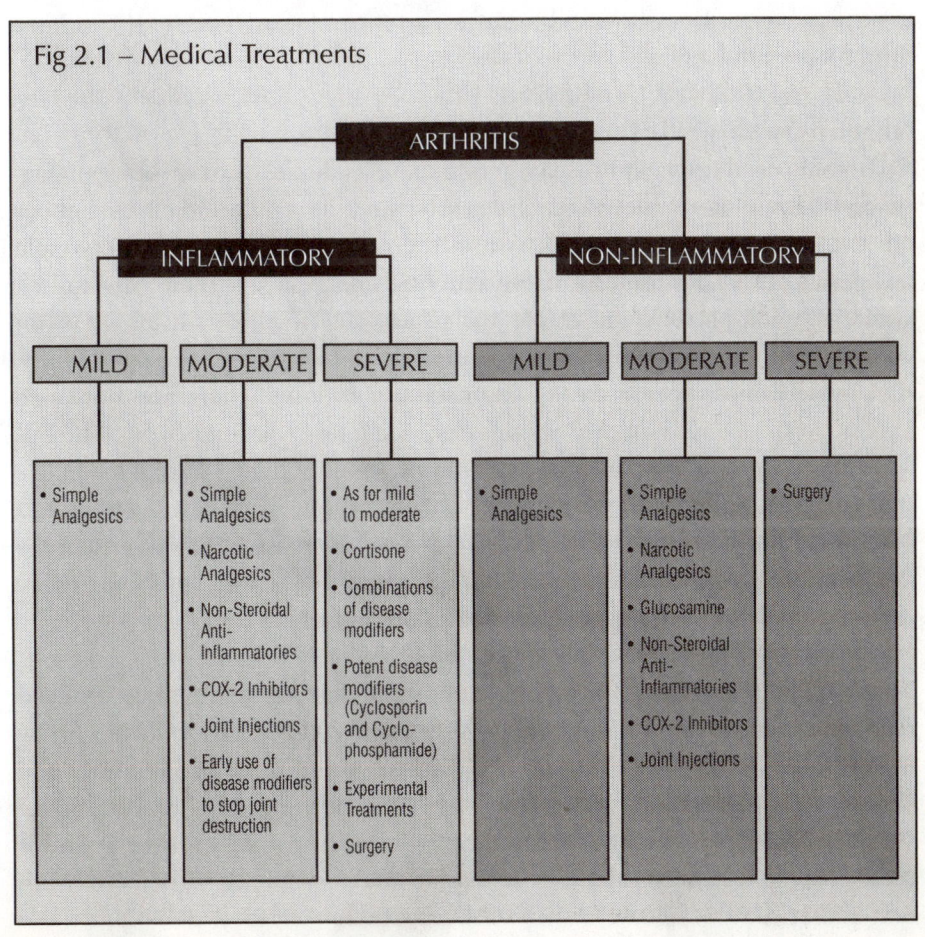

Fig 2.1 – Medical Treatments

DRUGS FOR SYMPTOM RELIEF

Drugs improve your life by either decreasing the pain or decreasing the inflammation of arthritis. They don't lead to suppression of the arthritis, and despite the fact you may be feeling more comfortable, it's possible a joint is still being damaged by your arthritis, which could led to deformity.

Simple analgesics

The only drug in this category is paracetamol (trade names include Panadol, Panamax, Dymadon). Paracetamol is a pure analgesic (pain killer) only. It has no effect on the arthritis itself, and is used for mild to moderate pain. The advantage of paracetamol is that it's not addictive and can be used at recommended doses for long periods. Most people tolerate it well and suffer few side effects. The disadvantages of paracetamol are that it's only a *mild* pain killer; and if you have kidney disease, use paracetamol in smaller doses — if you overuse it you run the risk of liver damage. You can take paracetamol orally by tablet or syrup formula, or rectally if you have difficulty swallowing.

Narcotic analgesics

Commonly used drugs in this category include codeine, dextropropoxyphene, oxycodone and morphine. These drugs are pain killers only and have no effect on the arthritis. You can safely use them in combination with simple analgesics. The advantage of using narcotic analgesics is their pain killing ability is much better than simple analgesics. The major disadvantage if you use them long term is they become addictive; and if you use them frequently, their effectiveness decreases and you need larger doses. There are more side effects from using narcotic analgesics, including dizziness, nausea and vomiting, constipation, abdominal cramps, euphoria and mood changes, nightmares, hallucinations, confusion, sedation, pinpoint pupils and sweating. Life-threatening side effects include a decrease in blood pressure, a decrease in heart rate and a decrease in breathing rate, although these extreme side effects are usually related to over-dosage.

Narcotic analgesics can be taken orally by tablets or syrups, by atomised face masks if in an inhaled form, rectally by suppository form, or by injection in either single doses or by infusion pumps over 24 hours. You should use narcotic analgesics sparingly (if at all) and only in acute flare-ups, until the pain has been brought under control with other types of medications. It is preferable to use simple analgesics long term as they are non-addictive.

Non-steroidal anti-inflammatory drugs

This group of drugs is used for mild to moderately severe arthritis. Non-steroidals are the most common arthritis drugs prescribed in the world. In the United States, some 70 million prescriptions are written annually, accounting for approximately 10 per cent of prescriptions worldwide. They are heavily prescribed for the elderly, and 20 per cent of all Australians over the age of 65 years use non-steroidals.

There are many different types in this group. While they may have different chemical compositions, they all act on the same chemical pathway involved in producing inflammation, and interfere with the production of the major inflammatory chemical, prostaglandin. They are very successful in decreasing arthritis pain, heat and swelling, but as a group they are idiosyncratic. One drug might be hopeless in decreasing your pain but another type might produce a brilliant response. Probably the most well known anti-inflammatory is aspirin, or salicylic acid. Others are naproxen, ibuprofen, indomethacin, piroxicam and diclofenac. Considering the number of people in the world who use these drugs, relatively few (5 to 7 per cent) have problems with non-steroidals. This means that more than 93 per cent of people can tolerate non-steroidals without a problem.

The major side effect with non-steroidals is that you might develop a stomach ulcer and the ulcer could start bleeding, as non-steroidals also thin the blood and decrease its clotting ability. You are at greater risk of a peptic ulcer while using non-steroidals if you are older, have a previous history of peptic ulcer and use oral cortisone at the same time as the non-steroidal. The longer-acting non-steroidals that are only taken once a day, such as piroxicam or ketoprofen, are also more likely to induce peptic ulceration compared with the shorter acting non-steroidals, such as diclofenac or ibuprofen. Gastroenterologists (stomach specialists) advise against using these drugs, but the alternatives are quite potent and have their own problems. There is not a better group of drugs available for treating mild to moderate arthritis than non-steroidals, although a new class of recently released drugs, cox-2 inhibitors (see below), will rapidly supersede non-steroidals as they don't induce stomach ulcers as commonly.

The other major problem with non-steroidals is their effect on the kidneys. When older people are admitted to hospital, routine blood tests often show a degree of kidney failure, which usually reverses when the non-steroidal is stopped. If you have previously had a stomach or peptic ulcer or if you have pre-existing kidney disease, don't use non-steroidals. Documented side effects with this group of drugs also include constipation, nausea, abdominal pain, dizziness, headache, itching, rash, tinnitus, shortness of breath and mouth ulcers. Less than 5 per cent of people experience these side effects, which means that most people can use them without safely.

WHILE NON-STEROIDAL DRUGS ARE THE MOST COMMONLY PRESCRIBED ARTHRITIS MEDICATION IN THE WORLD, A POTENTIAL SIDE EFFECT IS STOMACH ULCERS. YOUR DOCTOR WILL LET YOU KNOW IF THIS IS A POSSIBLE PROBLEM FOR YOU.

It's better to minimise non-steriodals—try to use them for acute flare-ups only. Using them in short bursts of up to a week when the arthritis is bad and then having some time off them can substantially decrease the risk of complications. Non-steroidal drugs can be given orally in tablet or syrup form, rectally by suppositories, by injection intramuscularly or by rubbing a gel or ointment over the skin of the joint. Whichever way you are given the non-steroidal, except with an ointment or gel, there is still the risk of stomach ulceration.

Cox-2 inhibitors

These drugs will eventually replace non-steroidal anti-inflammatory drugs because they are much less likely to cause stomach ulcers. In fact the incidence of this side effect with Cox-2 inhibitors is the same as someone taking placebo (sugar) tablets.

Cox-2 inhibitors work by inhibiting an enzyme called cyclo-oxygenase 2 (cox-2) which is involved in the production of inflammation and pain via the chemical prostaglandin. Cox-1 enzymes protect the stomach lining and non-steroidals inhibit both cox-1 and cox-2. This is why, as well as helping with inflammation, they also help produce stomach ulcers. Cox-2 only acts on the inflammation pathway and the stomach is left alone (see Figure 2.2). Cox-2 inhibitors also don't have any significant effect on the clotting of blood and there are apparently no bleeding problems if you take them. The cox-2 inhibitors are not disease-modifying drugs and are comparable to the older types of non-steroidal medications.

There are currently two cox-2 inhibitors on the market—Rofecoxib and Celecoxib. Therapeutically there is little difference between them. Because there is such a big market worldwide, other drug companies are likely to start producing them.

Possible side effects with cox-2 inhibitors are diarrhoea, headache, rhinitis, nausea and abdominal pain although the studies showed they were at the same levels as the adverse affects occurring with placebo medication (sugar tablets). If you have renal disease, be cautious using these drugs as they can affect the kidneys.

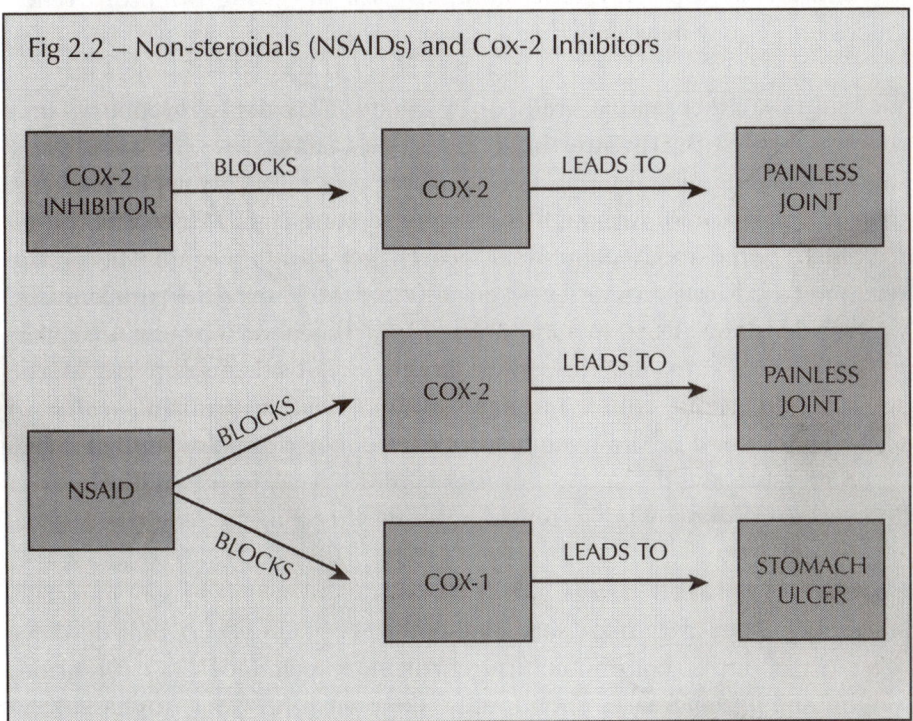

Fig 2.2 – Non-steroidals (NSAIDs) and Cox-2 Inhibitors

Glucosamine

Glucosamine is a recent naturopathic-based drug that in a series of small-scale studies with 20 to 30 patients has been found to give good symptom relief for people with osteoarthritis. It has also been confirmed by a much larger study of 1,200 patients in Portugal, which also showed the symptom relief and increased mobility lasted for up to 12 weeks after finishing the recommended course. As a result, glucosamine is beginning to be more accepted by the general medical community. However, one US study suggests that glucosamine is of no benefit for symptom relief of very advanced osteoarthritis, as the amount of cartilage remaining within the joint at this stage is minimal so the glucosamine has nothing to work on.

A compound naturally found in the cartilage of joints (glucosamine) is made from sugar (glucose) and an ammonia derivative (amine). One of its roles is to maintain the health of a joint and stop cartilage loss and the subsequent narrowing of the joint, a feature of osteoarthritis. As we age, the amount of glucosamine decreases as the amount of cartilage thins; treatment is aimed at improving the health and amount of cartilage present within the joint. Therefore, as well as giving symptom relief, glucosamine may help slow the disease process.

You can take glucosamine orally or by injection either intravenously, into the muscle, or directly into the joint. Studies suggest that people taking the intravenous glucosamine have a faster and more extensive response than to the placebo. Although the response starts more slowly than non-steroidals, after about eight weeks you'll get the maximum effect. The recommended oral dose is between 500 and 1000mg three times a day. Noticeable side effects include nausea, diarrhoea, indigestion and skin rashes. If you have diabetes, glucosamine may be inappropriate as the sugar component could increase your blood sugar. The salts of glucosamine used in the manufacture of the drug may also increase your blood pressure and if you use diuretics (fluid tablets) for heart disease and hypertension you may be better off avoiding this drug.

Cortisone-related drugs

Many people shy away from cortisone due to the side effects that develop. After two months' continuous use cortisone can induce fluid retention, weight and fat increase, thin fragile skin, easy bruising, higher blood pressure, mood changes, diabetes and osteoporosis. Prednisolone, prednisone, hydroxycortisone, methylprednisolone, betamethasone and triamcinolone are examples of cortisone-based drugs. You normally take them orally although they may also be given to you intravenously or injected directly into a joint.

Cortisol

Cortisone is actually made by the body in the form of cortisol. Cortisol is one of the body's steroids and is produced by the adrenal glands, which are located just above the kidneys in the abdomen. Cortisol has many different functions and is produced in just the right amounts by the adrenal glands so that your body is not overloaded with it and you don't get over-dosage side effects. As medicine, there is a fine line in the use of cortisol. The correct dose must be chosen that suppresses the disease without tending to give the myriad side effects possible with too large a dose.

The main role of cortisol in the body is the production of glucose in the liver. Cortisol stimulates the transport of amino acids from proteins in the skin, bone, muscle and connective tissue into liver cells. The result is a loss of protein in these cells but maximised glucose production in the liver. Glucose is the main fuel for cell metabolism and the only fuel that brain cells can use. When you exercise, experience a trauma, infection, anxiety and fever the adrenal glands respond within minutes. Your body under this sort of stress needs a higher fuel load — cortisol helps make sure you get enough glucose. Cortisol also:

▶ antagonises insulin action in the body, thereby increasing blood glucose levels for stressful situations
▶ regulates the body's water levels outside of cells
▶ regulates protein and fat metabolism in the body
▶ decreases the action of the immune system's white blood cells and their associated active chemicals
▶ acts as the body's natural anti-inflammatory.

Cortisol also reduces inflammation in the body (see Figure 2.3) by stabilising the membranes of lysosomes, little packages of enzymes within cells. Lysosomes are there to kill the cell if it is irreparably damaged by infection, or disease, or becomes worn out. Cortisol decreases the swelling of the inflammation by decreasing fluid leakage from small blood vessels. It does this by stabilising the blood vessel membrane and preventing other chemicals in the body, such as histamine, prostaglandins, interferon, lymphokines and bradykinine, from increasing the fluid content of tissues locally and thus adding to the inflammation. The fact that naturally occuring cortisol in the body has so many different functions is the reason why so many possible side effects can occur when it is administered therapeutically.

Unfortunately the use of cortisone in inflammatory arthritis is usually a long-term proposition, but with some types of arthritis cortisone is actually life-saving or can greatly improve quality of life. With cortisone the response is rapid and you will usually get relief within five to seven days of starting. Never use cortisone in septic (infective) arthritis. Septic arthritis should be absolutely excluded by your doctor before you use cortisone in any form. Cortisone switches off the body's natural immune system and if you already have an established infection, the infection can spread rapidly and aggressively.

If your arthritis is inflammatory in nature, cortisone is like a magic bullet and improves your quality of life immensely and quickly. So it's probably a waste of time using cortisone if you have osteoarthritis as there is minimal inflammation associated with this form and cortisone only works for inflammatory arthritis. Cortisone should only be used by people whose disease is of at least moderate severity where their lifestyle is greatly curtailed.

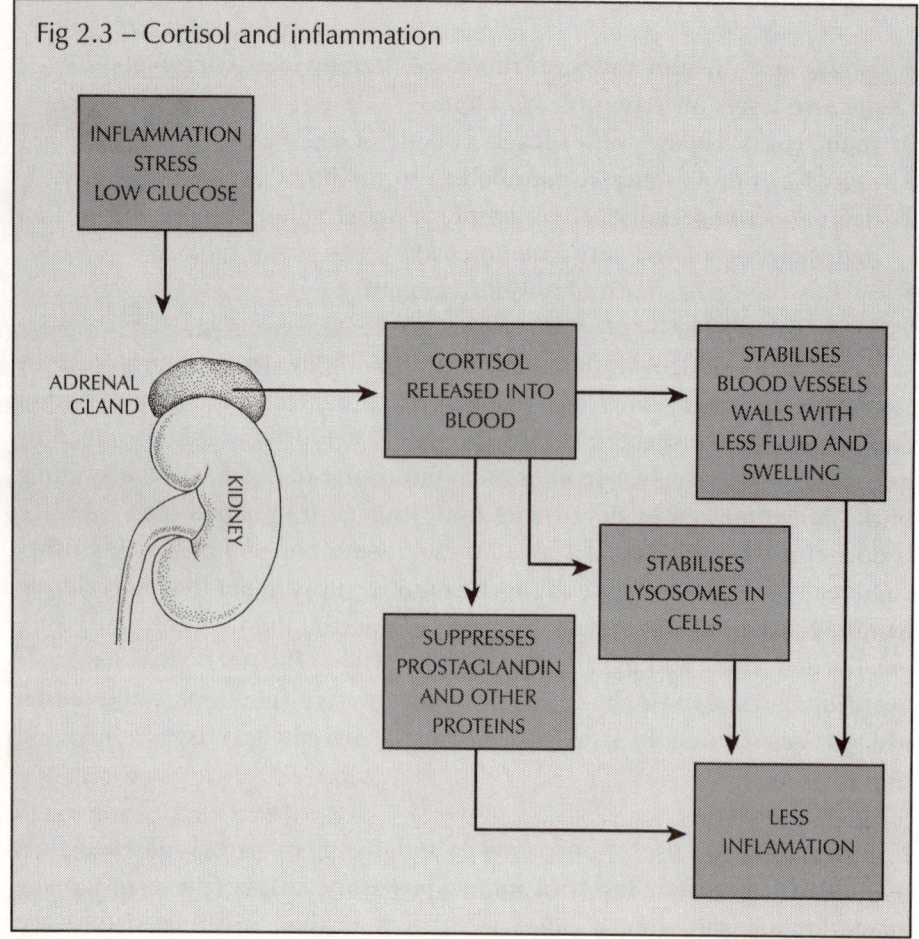

Fig 2.3 – Cortisol and inflammation

Once you begin cortisone treatment, don't stop it suddenly. It needs to be reduced in a controlled way for two reasons. First, when you are on oral cortisone, your body's production of cortisol tapers off to zero and the body relies on the dose that you swallow. If you stop taking the cortisone abruptly, the body takes a few days to restart production of natural cortisol. In the meantime the body is starved of cortisone and you can become sick. By slowly tapering off the dose, the body is able to gradually switch its cortisol production back on and meet the shortfall of the reducing dose. The second reason why you shouldn't stop cortisone overnight is the inflammatory arthritis becomes reliant on the cortisone for its suppression and when the cortisone is stopped suddenly, the arthritis rebounds and is usually more painful. Coming off cortisone is slow and may take several months.

Minimising the side effects of cortisone
To minimise side effects you can take cortisone in two ways—by pulse therapy and by joint injection. Pulse therapy is usually reserved for severe arthritis as it is very high dose and involves either two- or four-weekly doses of cortisone. These doses are usually 50 times the average daily dose and can be given orally or intravenously, although intravenous infusion usually means a day in hospital. As well as reducing arthritis inflammation, the side effects are much less than if you use the cortisone daily.

Joint injection, also known as intra-articular injection, sounds a painful way of getting treatment but if it's given by an experienced doctor, it shouldn't hurt any more than having a blood test. All joints, except the hip and spinal column joints, are easily accessible to injection, and if the cortisone is mixed with local anaesthetic at the same time, the result is immediate pain relief. I remember the morning of my wedding—my mother refused to come unless I did something about her painful arthritic shoulder. I did a quick injection into her shoulder joint with cortisone and local anaesthetic and 10 minutes later off we went.

The advantage of joint cortisone injections is that the cortisone only acts locally inside the joint and only very small amounts are absorbed from the joint into the rest of the body. So the side effect risk is minimised. You should not be given joint injections too frequently into the same joint and a maximum of four to six injections in one year is recommended. If the injections are too frequent a salt crystal of cortisone can develop inside the joint resulting in a painful flare-up of arthritis which mimics gout. Also too much steroid can damage the cartilage directly and worsen the arthritis. The risks associated with injection are bleeding into the joint and the introduction of infection into the joint via the needle. Both risks are very small.

THE USE OF CORTISONE IN INFLAMMATORY ARTHRITIS IS USUALLY A LONG-TERM OPTION.

Cortisone medications have a great deal to offer sufferers of inflammatory arthritis because they are highly effective in switching off the inflammatory reaction and giving you rapid symptom relief. This is especially so if you have a severe form and are unresponsive to non-steroidals although there is often a relapse when you stop. There is also now evidence suggesting cortisone will stop bone erosions developing in rheumatoid arthritis, indicating it has a role in supressing disease activity too. If your doctor prescribes cortisone drugs he or she may introduce a disease-modifying drug at the same time. Disease-modifying drugs take about three months to kick in and once they have, you can start weaning off the cortisone. You may then be able to rely on the disease-modifying drug alone or, at the very least, reduce the dose of cortisone which decreases the risk of side effects.

DISEASE-MODIFYING DRUGS
Appropriately named, these drugs do switch off the disease activity of an arthritis. As a group they are only suitable for inflammatory arthritis, having no effect on non-inflammatory types, and they definitely should not be used for osteoarthritis. They are very potent and some are used, in much higher doses, as chemotherapy for cancers. Ten years ago, these drugs would have been solely reserved for people with severe, destructive arthritis. Nowadays, the preference is to introduce these types of drugs much earlier and in less severe cases because they stop joint destruction. Rheumatologists also use combinations of these drugs because there is often a better response from using two or more drugs that have different mechanisms of action. By using combinations, you can use lower doses and minimise the risk of side effects while at the same time achieving better arthritis control.

The advantage of using a disease modifier over a long period of time is that the disease will be switched off, and there will be less joint destruction. There is less chance of developing side effects, in comparison to cortisone, and if your monitoring program is strictly adhered to, tests will pick up early abnormalities before you even notice them. The drug can then be stopped before any serious consequences develop.

Sulfasalazine

Also known as Salazopyrin, this drug is actually a combination of two drugs. One is a sulphur drug called sulfapyridine, which is an older type of antibiotic, and the other is salicylic acid, a non-steroidal anti-inflammatory called aspirin. Despite the fact that half the drug is a non-steroidal, there is more to its action than just the aspirin. Although how it works is still not fully understood, it does have an ability to interfere with lymphocyte (a white blood cell of the immune system) activity so that its production of immunoglobulins, leucotrienes and prostaglandin chemicals are altered, which results in decreased immune-originated inflammation. You can either take it orally or as a suppository.

Sulfasalazine is probably the best tolerated of the disease modifiers. It's usually used in moderate cases of arthritis or in combination with other medications and is the second most commonly used agent after methotrexate. Sulfasalazine is slow to act and it may take up to three months for you to notice any improvement. The dose is initially 500mg once daily and if tolerated over the next few weeks without any adverse reactions, and blood tests are normal, it is increased to 1000mg twice daily. However dosages up to 3000mg daily have been used.

Possible side effects are usually dose-related and can be alleviated by decreasing the dosage. Side effects include allergic reactions (especially to the sulfapyridine), gastrointestinal upset and nausea (although this can be minimised by using coated tablets), headaches, tinnitus, rashes, dizziness, pins and needles, breathing problems and infertility in men (which is reversible on stopping the drug). The more dangerous side effects from sulfasalazine are fortunately much less common. Especially important are the possible side effects on bone marrow and the liver, which may lead to anaemia, infections, bleeding and drug-induced hepatitis. This is why blood counts and kidney and liver tests must be done regularly when you're using sulfasalazine long term. It has been listed as safe to use in pregnancy with no proven adverse effects on the foetus.

Hydroxychloroquine

Also known as Plaquenil, nobody knows how hydroxychloroquine works but it is effective in treating systemic lupus erythematosus (also known as lupus) and rheumatoid arthritis. Also used to treat malaria, it's a cousin of quinine.

IF YOU ARE TAKING HYDROXYCHLOROQUINE, MAKE SURE YOU HAVE REGULAR EYE TESTS.

Hydroxychloroquine can only be taken in oral form and you may not notice any improvement in your arthritis for one to three months. The usual dosage is between 200mg and 400mg daily, taken in one dose. Always make sure you have a thorough eye examination before you take this drug, as it can damage both the corneas and retinas of the eyes through pigment deposits forming in these structures. An ophthalmologist can do computerised visual field tests and check the retina for defects. If the ophthalmologist gives the all clear it's a safe drug to use. Eye checks need to be repeated every six to 12 months and if you notice a change in vision while taking hydroxychloroquine tell your doctor immediately and stop taking the drug until the cause is found. Having said this, the problem is rare.

Other uncommon side effects of hydroxychloroquine are nausea, rashes and suppression of bone marrow. You will need to have periodic blood counts to monitor the bone marrow when taking this drug. Hydroxychloroquine is not recommended during pregnancy as it can cause neurological problems with the foetus.

Penicillamine

Although a breakdown product of the antibiotic penicillin, this drug has no antibiotic activity. There is ittle known about how penicillamine acts on inflammatory arthritis. The various possible explanations are that it interferes with the immune system, disrupts copper and zinc levels in the body thereby altering inflammation, interferes with the production of collagen for fibrous soft tissues of the joints, or has anti-viral activity. Whatever its action, it is a potent drug, but again it can still take up to three months to take maximum effect. The usual dosage is between 250mg to 750mg—to maximise absorption take it on an empty stomach. You also need to start on a low dose and gradually increase to your tolerance. Try taking it just before going to bed since it can give an annoying metallic taste and stomach upset which is not noticeable when you're sleeping. It can only be taken orally.

The other possible side effects are allergy reactions with rashes and itching, bone marrow suppression, kidney and liver dysfunction, mouth soreness, loss of collagen strength in the skin, iron deficiency and tinnitus. Don't take it if you're allergic to penicillin. Other side effects are uncommon. You will need to have regular blood tests to monitor bone marrow function, the occasional liver function test and urine to check for protein and blood. It should absolutely not be used during pregnancy.

Gold

The medical name for this drug is aurothioglucose and it was popular with rheumatologists in the 1970s and 1980s but has gone out of favour, probably because it has to be given by painful weekly to monthly injections. An oral tablet form was introduced but was much less effective than injections.

The action of gold on arthritis is not fully understood, but it appears to suppress the inflammation of the synovium of a joint associated with rheumatoid arthritis. It's not used in other forms of inflammatory arthritis except juvenile rheumatoid arthritis, also known as Still's Disease (see Chapter 7). Gold also appears to interfere with the action of immune cells and some of the chemicals associated with immune cells, such as histamine and prostaglandins. The response to gold in rheumatoid arthritis is a decrease in joint swelling, tenderness, pain and stiffness with an increase in grip strength. Gold is so effective in suppressing rheumatoid arthritis that British researchers have found gold wedding rings suppress the disease in the finger the ring is worn on and the adjacent finger joints are also less damaged. Apparently the gold is absorbed through the skin and into the local immune system of the joint, suppressing its action.

GOLD APPEARS TO HELP REDUCE THE INFLAMMATION OF ARTHRITIS. EVEN YOUR WEDDING BAND CAN SUPPRESS ARTHRITIS IN THAT FINGER AND ADJACENT FINGER JOINTS.

The usual strength of gold injections is at 50 per cent concentrations. The dosage schedule starts at 10mg with second and third doses of 25mg and fourth and following doses of 50mg. The doses are continued at weekly intervals until you have received approximately 1000mg. If your arthritis has improved and you haven't developed toxicity problems, the 50mg doses continue at four-weekly intervals and can continue for long periods of time—unless toxicity develops. Unfortunately it takes a cumulative dose of about 1000mg or about 20 weeks of treatment before you know if the gold has worked. Sometimes the dose can be decreased to 25mg depending on the response of the arthritis. Gold should never be used in pregnancy because foetal damage can occur.

It is not advisable to use hydroxychloroquine in combination with gold because of possible damage to the bone marrow. If you have diabetes, liver or kidney disease, heart failure, severe high blood pressure, lupus, Sjogren's syndrome or bleeding problems, you shouldn't use this combination.

If your gold use is properly monitored it's a safe drug and can be used for several years without a break. When gold was first introduced in rheumatology it was thought there was a maximum total dosage and when you got to that dose you couldn't use it any more. But the gold effect wore off and the arthritis returned. Gold is not a cure for inflammatory arthritis but does effectively switch the disease off while you're using it. Doctors don't worry about the total dose achieved and just monitor to make sure there are no problems developing.

The main worry with gold therapy is its effect on both the kidneys and the bone marrow. Before every gold injection your doctor should check your urine specimen to make sure there is no blood or protein in it, as these are indicators of kidney damage—unless another cause is found it's assumed this is due to gold. If blood and protein are present in your urine, you should abandon gold and have the cause and extent of kidney damage assessed. If the damage is caused by gold, the damage is almost always reversed when you stop the gold. Even if the damage is not due to gold, you should still abandon gold because it will make the damaged kidney worse.

To monitor the bone marrow, you will have routine blood counts one- to two-monthly. Again, changes to the bone marrow are mostly reversible on stopping gold. Other possible side effects induced by gold are itchy rashes, sore gums with or without mouth ulcers, and, rarely, nausea, gastrointestinal upset and eye inflammation. In the rare event of severe over-dosage of gold, you will be given another arthritis drug, penicillamine, to remove the excess from the body.

Gold in oral form, auranofin, is also available. The dosage is usually 6mg per day in adults. Oral gold has the same side effects as injected gold but

47 per cent of people using it complain of diarrhoea, 14 per cent complain of abdominal cramps and 10 per cent complain of nausea. Oral gold never seems to be as well tolerated or as effective as injected gold.

Methotrexate

Also known as methoblastin this drug was probably the arthritis drug of the 1990s. Methotrexate became popular with rheumatologists because it's a once-a-week oral dose and can give spectacular results within four to six weeks of starting it. This contrasts with other disease-modifying drugs, which can take three to six months to improve your symptoms. Methotrexate is extremely potent and it is a *once-a-week* dose *only*. The usual dose is somewhere between 10mg and 30mg per week, although most people end up on a dose around 15mg. It is potentially lethal to take it every day.

Methotrexate and the immune system

Methotrexate was first developed for chemotherapy for cancers. It works by stopping the genetic building blocks of cells, DNA, from replicating in cells. Because cancer cells have rapid cell production they need fast turnover of DNA to keep growing. If DNA production stops then the cancer does not grow. Methotrexate specifically stops DNA production by interfering with folic acid metabolism (see Figure 2.4). Folic acid is an essential mineral needed in cell function and reproduction. It's used in the production of bases of the amino acids purine and pyrimidine, and the conversion of serine to glycine. All of these amino acids are important in DNA synthesis. Folic acid is found in green leaf vegetables, liver and yeast.

The action of methotrexate in inflammatory arthritis relates to its action on rapidly dividing cells. The cells of the immune system also rapidly divide and replicate and because the methotrexate is not just specific for cancer cells, it can also affect other cells in the body.

The immune cells are very sensitive to the action of methotrexate and the result is a switching off of inflammation by decreasing immune cell numbers and function. It's a balancing act between switching the immune system off just enough to decrease the arthritis without switching it off so much that the immune system doesn't work at all. If the immune system is not working the body is susceptible to catching a major infection. The only way your doctor can make sure he or she is not overdoing it is by regular blood counts to assess bone marrow function. These are very

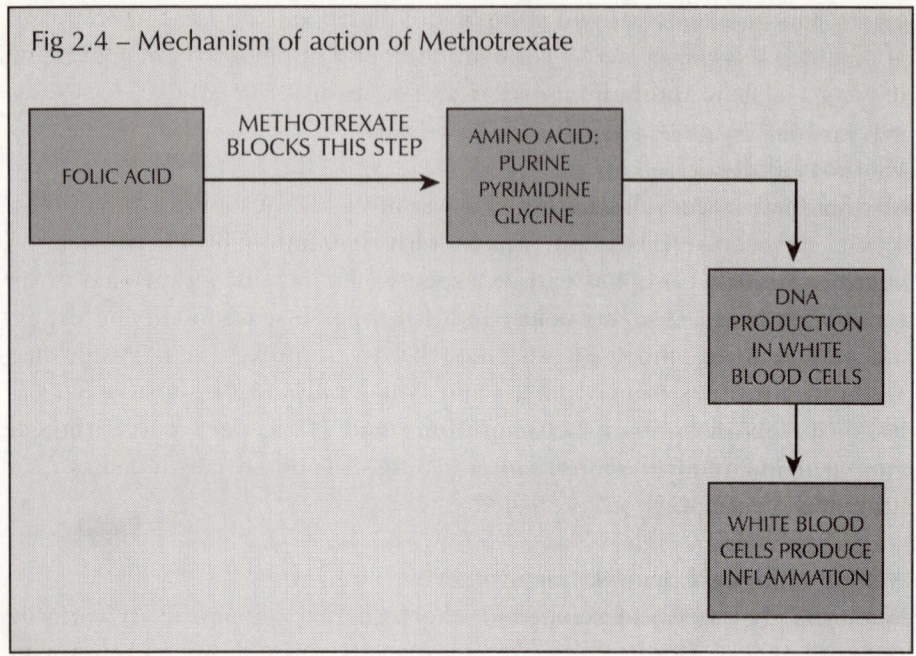

Fig 2.4 – Mechanism of action of Methotrexate

important and need to be done regularly. If there is a problem with the blood count, it usually comes back to normal on stopping the methotrexate.

The other major organ that needs regular monitoring is the liver as in a small number of people the liver can become cirrhotic. I have never seen this happen although I have stopped some patients' methotrexate treatment because they developed minor aberrations on liver function tests. All of these aberrations returned to normal upon stopping the drug. Patients did not feel that anything was wrong with their livers at the time. Methotrexate can also affect the lungs and kidneys but this is usually from the much higher doses used for cancer chemotherapy.

IF YOU'RE USING METHOTREXATE, YOUR DOCTOR NEEDS TO REGULARLY MONITOR YOUR BONE MARROW AND YOUR LIVER.

Other cells in the body that rapidly replicate can also be affected by methotrexate. Especially affected are the mouth and intestines with the possible result of mouth ulcers and stomach upset. Both of these side effects can usually be overcome by using supplemental folic acid of 5mg daily. Do not use methotrexate if you're pregnant or breastfeeding. It can affect both male and female fertility and is preferably used in people who have finished or don't intend having children. Some studies have also suggested that methotrexate can cause cancers because of its ability to damage the DNA in chromosomes, although this is mostly theoretical science and is rarely seen. Methotrexate should also never be used with salacylic acid or sulphonamide antibiotics—both these drugs increase the concentration of methotrexate in the blood, which may increase the risk of side effects.

There is no optimal duration for using a drug like methotrexate but it's likely to be at least six but preferably 12 months. There are only limited studies available on long-term methotrexate use and these indicate that improvement is maintained for at least two years with continual use. Some studies also suggest that when you stop methotrexate, a relapse of arthritis is possible within three to six weeks, although my experience is that it is much longer and some patients have gone into remission for several years. Whether this is due to the use of methotrexate or whether it would have occurred anyway I'm not sure.

Azathioprine

Also known as Imuran, azathioprine is converted in the body into 6-mercaptopurine, a substance similar to certain amino acids used in DNA synthesis. It is able to pass into cells and bind with other amino acids which form into DNA. As 6-mercaptopurine is not a true amino acid it interferes with DNA production, which leads to decreased cell reproduction, decreased cell numbers and less inflammation since the immune system cells are especially affected. With azathioprine these effects take up to three months before the patient notices a difference. The usual dosage is 50mg to 100mg daily taken orally, although higher doses are possible. You will usually be given cortisone as well to start with as the cortisone will give rapid relief of symptoms—when the azathioprine has become active you will be weaned off the cortisone.

In the doses used in rheumatology, side effects are relatively uncommon. Probably the worst reaction possible with azathioprine is an allergic hypersensitivity that can lead to malaise, headache, dizziness, vomiting, jaundice, pancreatitis, abnormal heart rhythms and heart failure. Fortunately this allergic reaction is rare and is reversible in the majority of cases when you stop the azathioprine.

Other possible side effects are bone marrow suppression, increased risk of infections, loss of hair and liver function disturbance. All these side effects are uncommon (occurring in fewer than 2 per cent of patients) and are reversible on stopping the azathioprine. Don't take azathioprine if you're pregnant as it can damage DNA during embryo development (pregnancy less than 12 weeks) and can lead to severe bone marrow suppression in the foetus (pregnancy greater than 12 weeks). Azathioprine interacts with a common gout drug called allopurinol—if they are used together the azathioprine dose should be a quarter of the normal dose as azathioprine clearance from the body is reduced by the allopurinol. You should have routine blood tests for bone marrow and liver function to monitor possible damage with azathioprine.

In rheumatology, azathioprine is used in rheumatoid arthritis, systemic lupus erythematosus (see Chapter 8), dermatomyositis (a disease that inflames the skin and muscles), and polymyositis (an autoimmune disease of the muscles).

Cyclophosphamide

This is a heavy duty drug used in arthritic conditions that are potentially life threatening, such as scleroderma, systemic lupus erethymatosus and primary Sjogrens syndrome. If the arthritis is going to shorten your life span it's reasonable to use a drug such as cyclophosphamide, as it not only increases your potential life expectancy, but also your quality of life. It has no role in mild to moderately severe arthritis because of its potential side effects.

Cyclophosphamide is a drug used in chemotherapy for cancers especially lymphomas, but it also has an important role in immune suppression, such as inflammatory arthritis. Cyclophosphamide itself is inactive but is converted by liver enzymes into active forms that interfere with immune cell reproduction and function. You would be given oral doses for arthritis up to 200mg daily, with the usual dose between 50mg to 100mg daily. Monitoring is essential with cyclophosphamide treatment because of its effect on the bone marrow with the possible result of severe infections, anaemia or bleeding problems. Usually this means a monthly blood count.

Other possible side effects include hair loss which is usually reversible on stopping the drug (but may result in a different hair colour growing back), inflammation of the bladder, allergic reactions, nausea and vomiting, diarrhoea, infertility in both males and females, lung inflammation, delayed wound healing and the development of some types of solid cancers. This last side effect is rare in rheumatology and usually occurs only if very high doses of cyclophosphamide are used. If you have had haemorrhagic inflammation of the bladder as a side effect of cyclophosphamide you are also at risk of developing cancer of the bladder several years later. This sounds awful but this drug would be a reasonable treatment option, despite the possible consequences, if the arthritis has affected your kidney, heart or lung, and you have been told your life expectancy is six months.

Cyclophosphamide also interacts with the gout medication allopurinol, and doses of cyclophosphamide should be decreased accordingly. Do not use cyclophosphamide if you are pregnant.

Cyclosporin

This is a combination of amino acids produced by the fungus *tolypocladium inflatum gams*. It's a very powerful immune suppressive drug that has revolutionised the transplantation of the kidney, heart, lungs and pancreas. Immunosuppression is important in inflammatory arthritis, especially in rheumatoid arthritis and psoriasis-induced arthritis (see Chapter 12) where the white blood cells (lymphocytes) are especially affected in their production of inflammatory chemicals. Like cyclophosphamide its use is restricted to severe forms of arthritis. Unlike other potent immunosuppressives it doesn't affect the bone marrow and there is less likelihood of anaemia, infections and bleeding problems.

Like most disease-modifying drugs, cyclosporin is slow in its action on arthritis, however if you don't have a response in six months you should stop taking it.

There is no set dose of cyclosporin. Your doctor will determine the dose based on blood tests showing the concentration of cyclosporin in your blood. This varies from person to person due to levels of absorption of the drug from the gut, how it is distributed throughout the body organs, and how quickly it is eliminated from the body via the liver. Don't use cyclosporin if you have underlying liver or kidney problems, cancers or pre-cancers present (including skin cancers), uncontrolled high blood pressure, infections or any serious heart disorders. In general the doses used in rheumatology are much lower than those used in its other main use, organ transplantation, so the risk of side effects is decreased. You take cyclosporin daily in oral tablet form.

Cyclosporin has the potential for serious side effects. If you're taking cyclosporin you'll need to have regular routine monitoring which should include blood pressure, urine examination for protein and blood tests for cyclosporin levels, blood counts, kidney and liver function and electrolyte levels, especially potassium. You'll probably find your blood pressure goes up when on cyclosporin, but anti-hypertension medications are usually enough to control this problem. High potassium levels in the blood are potentially lethal as they could induce abnormal heart rhythms but it is reversible and can settle spontaneously. It's best to avoid foods high in potassium, such as bananas, when using cyclosporin.

IF YOU'RE TAKING CYCLOSPORIN, YOUR BLOOD PRESSURE WILL PROBABLY GO UP. YOUR DOCTOR WILL MONITOR THIS AND PRESCRIBE ANTI-HYPERTENSION MEDICATION IF NECESSARY.

Cyclosporin can also lead to increased cholesterol levels, decreased blood magnesium levels, decreased vaccination levels from immunisations and make you more at risk of gout. Less common side effects include excess hair growth, fluid retention, diarrhoea, skin rashes, headaches, hearing loss, convulsions, pins and needles, increased blood sugar levels, cramps and muscle weakness. Cyclosporin also may increase the risk of a lymphoma cancer developing.

Take care using cyclosporin if you're using other drugs at the same time because the levels of both cyclosporin and the other drug may go up or down depending on the interaction between the drugs. Some drug interactions have been proven, but many are only suspected. The safe thing to do would be to check the cyclosporin blood level after starting the new drug to make sure there has been no change in blood levels.

Leflunomide
Leflunomide is metabolised in the body to its active component, an isoxazole, which inhibits the action of an enzyme involved in the synthesis of pyrimidine. Pyrimidine is an essential chemical used in energy pathways in cells and in production of DNA and RNA in cells. This action leads to immune system suppression. When used in rheumatoid arthritis it was found to be effective within four weeks of its use and it apparently was as

effective as sulfasalazine, gold, methotrexate and cyclosporin. You take leflunomide orally and it lasts a long time in the body. The usual starting dose is 100mg for the first three days followed by a maintenance dose of 10 to 20mg daily.

Don't use leflunomide if you have a pre-existing liver disease as it can cause problems with liver function. The liver abnormality is generally reversible on stopping the drug. You should have monthly liver function blood tests to monitor the leflunomide. Most people tolerate the drug well but side effects could include loss of appetite, nausea, abdominal pain, diarrhoea, hypertension, dizziness, hair loss and inflammation of the lungs. I find the biggest problem with it is the diarrhoea and have had to suspend its use in about one in four cases due to this side effect.

---

*IF YOU HAVE ANY PROBLEMS WITH YOUR LIVER,
YOU SHOULD NOT TAKE LEFLUNOMIDE.*

Leflunomide can cause genetic damage to the embryo in pregnancy so if you're a woman planning a pregnancy don't take leflunomide. The manufacturer of the drug goes so far as to recommend you use contraception while you're taking the drug. It can also genetically damage spermatozoa in men. If you're planning a pregnancy you should have a wash out procedure done to eliminate the drug from the body as leflunomide can last for up to two years in the body's tissues. It is recommended for both men and women and is simply done by swallowing recommended doses of either cholestyramine or charcoal for 11 days.

Conclusion

There is a reasonable choice of disease-modifying drugs available for treatment of inflammatory arthritis (see Figure 2.5). The treatment regimes vary and, depending on your circumstances, some are more suitable than others. All disease modifiers are potent and have potential for side effects. There are risks using these drugs and the benefits must outweigh the risks for you to start using them. The risks of these drugs are diminished substantially if they are monitored appropriately and it's extremely important that the doctor prescribing these drugs is familiar with and experienced in their use. Ask your doctor about his or her experience in using them before you agree to take them, and ask your

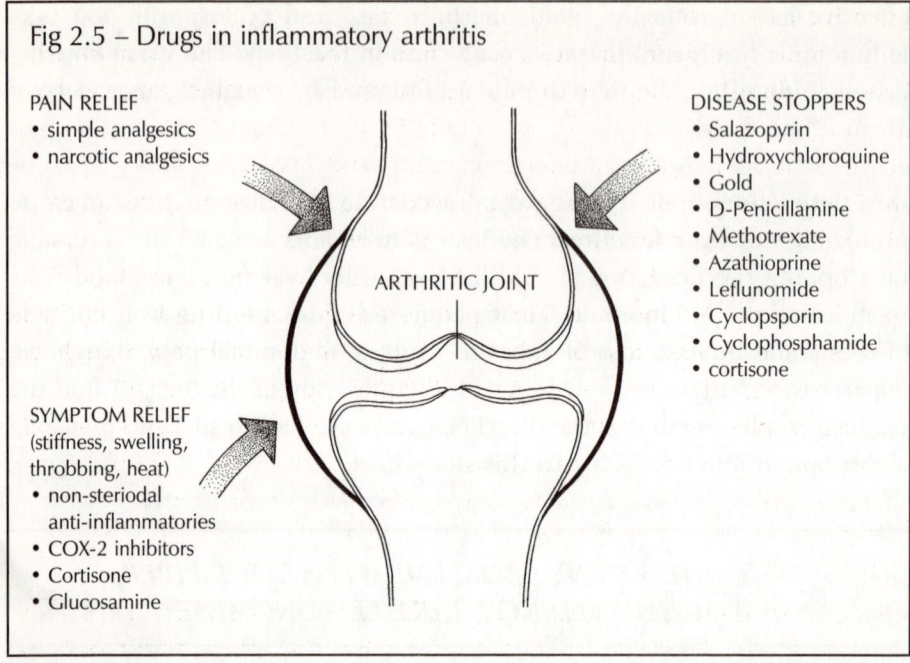

Fig 2.5 – Drugs in inflammatory arthritis

PAIN RELIEF
• simple analgesics
• narcotic analgesics

DISEASE STOPPERS
• Salazopyrin
• Hydroxychloroquine
• Gold
• D-Penicillamine
• Methotrexate
• Azathioprine
• Leflunomide
• Cyclopsporin
• Cyclophosphamide
• cortisone

ARTHRITIC JOINT

SYMPTOM RELIEF
(stiffness, swelling, throbbing, heat)
• non-steriodal anti-inflammatories
• COX-2 inhibitors
• Cortisone
• Glucosamine

specialist to notify your family doctor about the monitoring regimes needed to use the drugs safely. These drugs can greatly improve your quality of life, so don't be afraid to use them.

*SOME OF THE NEWER ARTHRITIS DRUGS
ARE STILL IN THE EXPERIMENTAL PHASE.*

FUTURE DRUGS

There are certain new drugs about to be released or that have recently been released. Health professionals have limited familiarity with these drugs and any potentially serious side effects may not be known until larger populations of patients have taken them. For example, one drug called Etanercept has now been shown to increase the risk of serious infections. This was not known or reported in the original studies or press releases and did not come to light until after it was fully approved by American drug regulatory authorities. These new drugs are also expensive and the cost versus benefit needs to be explored before their release. The recently released leflunomide, for example, is $A4500 per patient per year compared with methotrexate which is approximately $A200 per patient per year. The new injected tumour necrosis factor related drugs cost aproximately $18,000 per year.

Etanercept

This new drug, a recombinant human tumour necrosis factor receptor p75: Fc fusion protein, attempts to block inflammation via pathways that have not been previously explored. By blocking a particular receptor of human necrosis factor on cell surfaces, inflammation decreases. It has worked in rheumatoid arthritis patients who have not responded to prior therapy with azathioprine, methotrexate or penicillamine.

You take etanercept via twice weekly injections. In studies to date, patients were injected for six months with 50 to 60 per cent showing significant improvements in their rheumatoid arthritis. The studies suggested that etanercept was well tolerated with mild injection site reactions the only significant side effect. Because etanercept increases risk of infection, it now carries warnings for its use and should not be used if you have an infection.

Infliximab

Also called Remicade, infliximab is another new drug that targets the human protein, tumour necrosis factor, which is involved in the production of inflammation in rheumatoid arthritis. Infliximab doesn't bind or block the receptor site on the cell surface but actually binds to the tumour necrosis factor, enlarging the molecule so that it's physically too big to bind to its active site on the cell wall, thereby making the tumour necrosis factor inactive.

You take infliximab by intravenous infusion about six to eight times a year. The logistics of arranging this and the actual cost of the drug make this drug particularly expensive. The manufacturer recommends you take another disease-modifying drug at the same time, such as methotrexate. About half the people who took infliximab claimed a 20 to 30 per cent improvement in lifestyle and about two-thirds of people experienced decreased joint tenderness and swelling.

Side effects with infliximab are reported as mild and include headaches, nausea, sinusitis and rashes. Like etanercept it may affect your immune system's ability to fight infections and you probably shouldn't take it if you have an infection.

Tacrolimus

This drug is used to suppress the immune system after an organ or bone marrow transplant and, like cyclosporin, may suppress the immune system in rheumatoid arthritis. A very small study of 12 people with severe rheumatoid arthritis who had failed to respond to treatment with other disease-modifying drugs, were given tacrolimus with the majority showing improvement in their condition. However there was a high dropout due to side effects of upset stomach, chest pain and neuralgia pain so its use will be limited to severe disease in which other drugs have failed.

Nitric oxide combined with non-steroidals

Still in the experimental arena, the theory is that the nitric oxide protects the lining of the stomach, while the non-steroidal acts against inflammation, thereby minimising the risk of stomach ulcers caused by the non-steroidal-induced prostaglandin deficiency. Nitric oxide/non-steroidal combinations are predicted by some health professionals to supersede cox-2 inhibitors because they maintain the benefits of cox-1 inhibition from non-steroidals, such as protection against heart attacks and the decreased incidence of bowel cancer when using aspirin.

Other ideas

One of the most exciting future developments is vaccinations for different types of arthritis. Obviously we need to find out if an infection causes the arthritis before it can be immunised against—researchers worldwide are trying to identify infective agents with the hope of a breakthrough.

Another possible type of vaccination is one that 'switches off' the part of the immune system that is stimulating the inflammation within a joint, or neutralises the chemicals involved. A vaccine for the inflammation of rheumatoid arthritis has recently been developed in the United States. In a very small trial, a 70 per cent response rate has been claimed. Bigger trials will show how successful this will be.

In the United States, the Food and Drug Authority has given the green light for the use of a blood filtering machine to be used in the treatment of rheumatoid arthritis. This is similar to kidney dialysis, where a machine is used to filter toxins out of the body of a person with kidney failure. In rheumatoid arthritis, the theory is that the machine filters out all the 'bad' proteins involved in inducing inflammation, and with smaller loads of inflammatory proteins in the body the disease will be less active. One possible drawback is it's a costly machine to buy and operate. Also, you need to have a needle inserted into your vein to filter the blood and the more often you have the procedure done, the more difficult (and painful) it is to get access to your veins. Sterility is essential so that no infections are introduced into the patient's body and because of this blood filters will probably only be used for severe cases of inflammatory arthritis.

SURGICAL TREATMENTS

Surgical treatments are continually improving and can successfully relieve symptoms or improve the functioning of a joint. The most common joint surgery relating to arthritic conditions is a joint replacement. Hips and knees are the most common joint replacements, so much so that they have become routine surgery for most orthopaedic surgeons. Surgeons can also replace shoulder joints, knuckle joints in the hands, joints between the feet and toes and elbows. If you need to have these other joint replacements, make sure you choose a surgeon experienced in this area. Post-surgical care is important and you might need splints with pulley systems to improve functioning during the healing process—especially if you've had a hand joint replaced.

SURGERY CAN RELIEVE ARTHRITIC SYMPTOMS
AND IMPROVE THE FUNCTIONING OF A JOINT.

Joint surgery may be appropriate if the joint function is impaired. The different effects of rheumatoid arthritis can provide a good example. Even though you may have a major deformity to your hand, your hand may still function adequately and be able to manipulate fine objects: if your hand functions well there is no point doing major joint replacement of the hand. If, however, you have difficulty manipulating small objects you are better off having the deformity fixed. With rheumatoid arthritis the heads of the knuckles are excised off and replaced with silastic cups. Silastic is a flexible plastic compound, similar to the silicone used to waterproof cracks in a bathroom. It allows for straightening of the joint and improves functioning.

Other types of surgery possible in rheumatoid arthritis include tendon reconstruction to correct tendon rupture and malalignment, and arthrodesis (fixing) of the joint of the base of the thumb to stabilise the joint, improve functioning of the thumb and provide pain relief. Wrist deformities in rheumatoid arthritis can be fixed either by arthrodesis or silastic joint replacement. You can also have similar reconstructive surgery for foot deformities.

Fig 2.6 – A total knee replacement

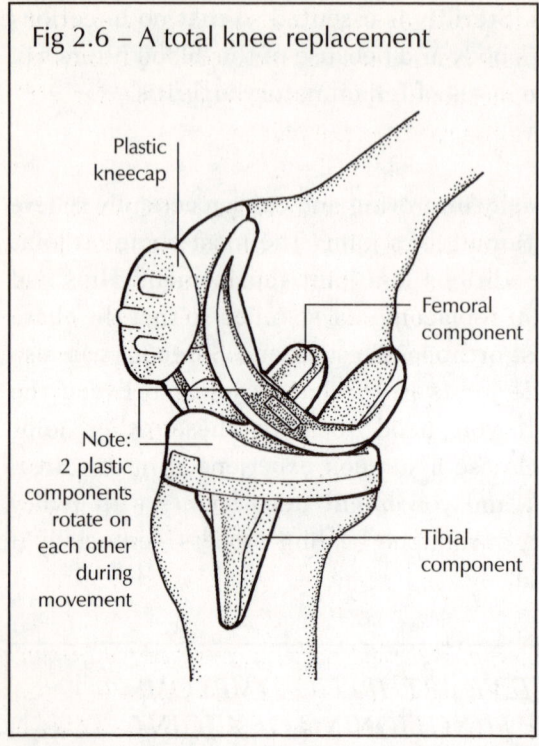

Plastic
kneecap

Femoral
component

Note:
2 plastic
components
rotate on
each other
during
movement

Tibial
component

Fig 2.7 – A total hip replacement

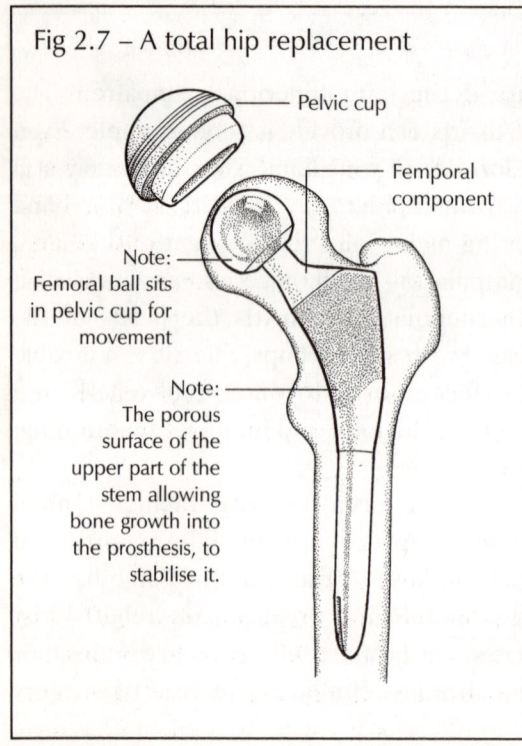

Pelvic cup

Femoral
component

Note:
Femoral ball sits
in pelvic cup for
movement

Note:
The porous
surface of the
upper part of the
stem allowing
bone growth into
the prosthesis, to
stabilise it.

Hip and knee replacements

Osteoarthritis is the usual reason you would have a hip or knee replacement (see Figures 2.6 and 2.7). Both procedures are highly successful in most people. If you suffer from osteoarthritis, you know how unbearable the pain can be and how your mobility can be affected. Osteoarthritis can lead to deformity and result in decreased functioning of the joint, especially in the knee, which is bowed outwards. This deformity is another criteria for joint replacement.

In hip replacements, you would normally have both halves of the joint replaced. The hip is a ball and socket joint and in hip joint replacement the head of the femur (thigh bone) is the ball; this is replaced with a metal ball on a stalk, and the pelvic acetabulum (pelvic cup) is replaced with a plastic cup. The femoral component is made of either stainless steel, titanium or a cobalt-chrome alloy. The pelvic component is made of either high-density polyethylene plastic or a ceramic mixture. The ceramic cup is less well thought of despite having better frictionless characteristics because it's more easily broken. The type of prosthetic component your surgeon chooses depends on which one he or she is most comfortable using, since there are over 300 prosthetic components available for hip replacements alone.

The two prostheses can either be cemented into position with an acrylic cement called methylmethacrylate or can be placed into position and fixed by new bone growing through holes in the surfaces of the prosthesis. The advantage to cementing is that it fixes the prosthesis rapidly allowing the patient to mobilise and bear weight faster; the drawback is the cemented joint doesn't generally last as long. As a rough guide cemented joints last about 10 years before needing to be replaced and non-cemented, bone fixed joints last about 15 years before wearing out. So joint replacement tends to be restricted to patients who are over 60 so that surgery is likely to be limited to once only. However it may also be the best option in a young patient otherwise confined to a wheelchair.

If a non-cemented joint is put in, you will be on crutches for much longer and won't be able to bear weight until the bone grows into the prosthesis, which can take six to 10 weeks. Although recovery is slower, you will have a longer-life joint replacement.

Infection
One of the major concerns with joint replacement is infection, which means the components and surrounding damaged bone need to be removed. Even with intravenous and oral antibiotics, it takes weeks for the infection to be overcome. It's then extremely difficult for a new replacement to be put in. For this reason, surgeons who do joint replacements use strict anti-infection measures such as:

▶ special ultra-clean air operating theatres where the air is pumped out of the operating room to prevent any germs entering the theatre
▶ giving antibiotics before, during and after surgery
▶ antibiotic laden cement.

I remember one of my first terms as an intern in orthopaedic surgery. Part of my job was to check the patients over before they had surgery. I had to make sure they were totally infection free and healthy enough for surgery. I thoroughly examined one patient the evening before surgery, especially checking the hip to make sure there was no skin infection. The next morning I copped an almighty mouthful from my boss, because the patient had grown a small pimple at his operation site overnight, and we didn't find out his hip was contaminated until we had fully anaesthetised and paralysed him for the operation! Unfortunately the anaesthetist had to wait around for 90 minutes for the anaesthetic to wear off and the patient had an extra anaesthetic because we had to get him back in a week later once the pimple had disappeared.

Hip replacement is major surgery and is often done if you're older or have other complicating diseases. These increase the risk of surgery and anaesthesia, although the anaesthetic risk can be minimised if only a spinal or regional anaesthetic is used. Other risks include deep vein thrombosis, infection, fracture of the surrounding bone structures (especially if the bone is osteoporotic), damage to the surrounding nerve structure (such as the sciatic nerve in hip replacements), loosening of the hip joint with time (usually due to poor cementing), and excess bone formation around the replaced joint which interferes with functioning and mobility. Joint replacements are nevertheless successful overall.

ALTHOUGH THERE ARE SOME RISKS ASSOCIATED WITH SURGERY, JOINT REPLACEMENTS ARE USUALLY VERY SUCCESSFUL. HIP AND KNEE REPLACEMENTS ARE THE MOST COMMON JOINTS TO BE REPLACED.

Knee replacements are also a common joint replacement, particularly if you have osteoarthritis or rheumatoid arthritis. The femoral (thigh bone) prosthetic component is usually metallic and the tibial (shin bone) component is usually a metal backed polyethylene table on which the femoral component rotates with joint movement. The knee joint has three compartments and if only one compartment is affected by arthritis you can have a unicompartment replacement as an alternative. This procedure has superseded the older tibial wedge osteotomy where the surgeon cuts a wedge of bone out of the shin bone in a bowed knee, which leads to straightening of the knee. The knee might be straightened with the osteotomy but there is no improvement to the arthritis and eventually you would need a knee replacement.

Knee replacements are now as successful as hip replacements—you can expect a cemented knee joint to last 10 or more years. The complications of knee replacements are the same as for hip replacements and, as for hip replacements, there are arguments for both cemented and non-cemented knee replacements.

Replacing the Shoulder Joint

Joint replacement of the shoulder is also possible in osteoarthritis and rheumatoid arthritis. The success of this operation depends on the integrity of surrounding soft tissue such as ligaments, tendons and muscles. If your arthritis has severely damaged these structures you will get significant pain relief from this operation although your mobility won't be improved much.

HYALURONAN INJECTIONS

Hyaluronan is a mucopolysaccharide (mucus = protein, poly = many, saccharide = sugar) that occurs naturally in the synovial fluid of a joint and is the substance that makes the fluid treacle-like, giving the joint fluid good elasticity and viscosity. Hyaluronan also occurs in the cartilage of a joint. One of the functions of synovial fluid in a joint is to help lubricate the joint and decrease internal friction when the joint moves.

If you have osteoarthritis, there is both a loss of cartilage and loss of hyaluronan within the joint. Surgeons don't routinely replace cartilage yet (although cartilage grafts are technically feasible) but can now replace the loss of hyaluronan with hylans (the trade name is Synvisc), a synthetically produced component of hyaluronans. Hylans is simply injected directly into a joint to replace or supplement the loss of hyaluronan. This improves lubrication of the joint and also acts as a shock absorber for it. Hylans is only recommended for osteoarthritis as this disease leads predominantly to cartilage and joint degeneration with loss of hyaluronan. It is not a cure for osteoarthritis as it is only replacing lost substances, but the improvement in the joint lasts about six months. In severe osteoarthritis, hylans may delay the inevitable surgery you need by relieving your pain.

The usual treatment regime for hylans is three injections spaced one week apart. Because hylans is a semi-natural product, your body metabolises it over time—this is why you need repeat injections. Theoretically any joint with osteoarthritis is amenable to treatment with hylans, except the hip and spinal joints as they are too difficult to routinely access with a needle. Currently the major recommendation from the manufacturer of hylans is for osteoarthritis of the knee. You may gain relief after one injection but most people feel the full benefit about five to nine weeks after the third injection. If after six months the improvement wears off you can repeat the course of three injections.

Because hylans is not a drug as such there are no chemical reactions and it acts physically within the joint to supplement what's damaged or missing. The manufacturers of hylans claim a small percentage of people who have the hylans injection may have short-lived, local discomfort or swelling in the joint. An allergic reaction to hylans is also possible.

The downside of hylans treatment is the cost of approximately $200 per injection with no government rebate through Medicare or the pharmaceutical benefits scheme.

ALLIED HEALTH TREATMENTS
Many rheumatology units have allied health specialists—physiotherapists, hydrotherapists, occupational therapists and podiatrists.

Physiotherapy
You can have physiotherapy if you have an acute arthritic attack—some of the techniques used will decrease swelling and pain and also improve circulation to the joint to aid healing. Physiotherapists also use ultrasound (high frequency sound waves) and inferential stimulation to improve blood flow to the joint and surrounding soft tissues. With inferential stimulation an electrical current is sent through the tissues which, as well as promoting healing, switches off the surrounding pain fibres. This is similar to a TENS machine (transcutaneous electrical nerve stimulator) used to relieve chronic pain. Several electrode pads are placed around your spine or damaged area and a small current is run through it. Your skin tingles when the machine is switched on and the current is gently increased to affect the nerve fibres.

Physiotherapy is essential if you have chronic arthritis because it improves the range of movement of the joint. The greater the range of movement, the greater the mobility and function of the joint.

Hydrotherapy
Hydrotherapy can be used with physiotherapy—your joints are weightless in water so the movements are less stressful. The other advantage of hydrotherapy is that you're usually part of a group which is often a good

motivator. You can continue physiotherapy and hydrotherapy exercise regimes long term and, once learned, at a time convenient for you. Both physiotherapy and hydrotherapy usually concentrate on the large joints of the body.

PHYSIOTHERAPY AND HYDROTHERAPY CAN HELP YOU MANAGE YOUR ARTHRITIS.

Occupational therapy

Occupational therapy aims to improve your fine motor ability, in particular manipulation of small objects. For this reason occupational therapists usually concentrate on the hands. As well as helping hand function, occupational therapists make hand splints and braces that improve the positioning of joints both at rest and with use. These are important because abnormal directional forces act on joints when they are deformed, and the joints worsen with use. Occupational therapists can give you gadgets for everyday use to decrease the amount of force needed in a hand action, or to help you with manipulative movements. For example, knives and forks can be designed especially for arthritic hands, or a leverage gadget to help you turn on taps. The arthritis association in your state can also tell you where to get these devices.

IF YOU HAVE BADLY ARTHRITIC HANDS, AN OCCUPATIONAL THERAPIST CAN GIVE YOU GADGETS TO HELP YOU WITH PARTICULARLY DIFFICULT TASKS.

Podiatry

Podiatrists specialise in feet. If you have arthritis, you may find it difficult to bend over far enough to cut your toenails, or find that your hands may be too arthritic to hold a toenail clipper. Some types of arthritis, such as rheumatoid arthritis and scleroderma, are associated with damage to the blood supply to the feet, which can result in an increased risk of foot infection. Also if the nerve doesn't have an adequate blood supply you can get nerve damage. This means your feet can lose their sensation to pain, cold and heat, making them more susceptible to trauma and injury, and affecting balance (some balance receptors are located in the joints of the feet). A good podiatrist will assess and monitor this problem.

If your feet are deformed by arthritis you'll get secondary damage from the abnormal walk that develops. This can put abnormal forces on the joint, which then worsens the whole problem. A podiatrist can help by manufacturing special shoe inserts or special shoes that fit the dynamics of your arthritic walk and take the stresses off the joints.

HELP WITH DAILY LIVING

The symptoms of arthritis can make it difficult to do normal everyday things. Such mundane actions as turning the tap on, going to the toilet, dressing, cooking or doing the housework become more than just a simple chore—they can become downright impossible. However there are ways that you can minimise these problems.

Bending

If your electric sockets are at floor level get them relocated to waist level so that you don't have to bend down to reach them. You can also do this with other objects around the house or use tongs to pick up low-lying objects to minimise bending.

Slipping

Make floor surfaces safe so that there's no chance you'll slip over. Highly polished floors might look good, but they make a hard landing place. Floor coverings, such as carpets, should be firmly stuck to the floor—loose rugs are also a tripping hazard. Lighting needs to be bright enough to prevent you tripping.

Opening doors

Opening a door with a round doorknob is extremely difficult for an arthritic hand. Install lever-type door handles and get a locksmith to modify door keys to give a better grip.

Stairs

The ultimate solution with stairs is to move into a home without them. If this isn't possible, install a second handrail on the wall opposite the banister to give you extra support and security. Make sure the stair surface is not slippery, that the stair carpet is firmly fixed down and that stair lighting is good. Stair lifts are an expensive option.

Bathrooms

Taps, like round doorknobs, can be difficult to use, so install lever taps, which are readily available and easy to use. For the bath and shower, handrails are an essential safety feature. Use a seat in the bath or shower to avoid falling over on a slippery, wet surface. Non-slip surfaces such as rubber bathmats may also help. Look for washing implements that are easy to use, such as scarf-like wash cloths for washing your back, long-handled body brushes, washing mittens, and soap on a string. Handrails can also help with access to the toilet. Foot operated flushes or even self-flushing systems may be easier for you to use than small levers or buttons. High-level toilet seats are also available.

Kitchens

Make sure your kitchen surfaces and shelves are all at the right height, as this optimises your posture and limits bending over. You can either install a new kitchen or go for the cheaper option and find a raised, high-backed chair so that you don't have to stand all the time. Try to keep the kitchen compact, with close working surfaces, so that you can slide pots and pans (preferably lightweight pans) rather than carry them. Put lever taps in the sink and check whether you can modify the knobs on the stove-top. Choose the refrigerator with care—those with a freezer at the bottom might be more practical as you visit the fridge more often than the freezer. Use electric can openers and devices fixed to the wall to give leverage in opening jar lids.

Eating

If you have a poor grip use two hands instead of one for picking up cups and preferably use light, insulated cups. Forks, spoons and knives with thick handles improve grip.

Dressing

Dressing sticks with a hooked end for pulling clothes on and a rubber-tipped end for pushing clothes off will help enormously. Buttons and shoelaces can be a problem so buy clothes with velcro strips and slip-on shoes.

Cleaning and housework

If you can afford it, employ someone to clean for you. Use appliances with large electric plugs to make insertion and removal into power sockets easier. Using long handled dustpans and brushes allows you to sweep without bending over, and lightweight carpet sweepers put less stress on the body than heavy vacuum cleaners. Fitted bed covers and sheets along with doonas/duvets are much easier to put on and off the bed.

Cars

If you can, get a car with power steering, and consider installing wide-angled mirrors so that you don't have to twist your spine as much to check over your shoulder. Easy reach seat belts can also limit twisting.

Gardening

Many tools have been designed for arthritic conditions and finding the ones that suit you involves research and a bit of trial and error. Tools that maximise leverage and minimise the effort you put in are the best ones. You can get ratchet-action branch cutters, various long-handled grabbers and weeders, wheel rakes, hoes, electric trimmers and motorised mowers and edge cutters. Minimise bending and lifting by planting in pots and in raised steel and fibreglass beds.

COMPLEMENTARY TREATMENTS

C omplementary therapies provide genuine relief to many people. It's unfortunate that some members of the medical fraternity don't believe in these treatments and that some complementary practitioners bypass medical science. The main objective of all health practitioners, whatever their discipline, is to help your suffering. Although my preference is for medical therapies, if a complementary therapy works for you, embrace it. However it is important to check that therapists are registered practioners in their field.

MASSAGE

Massage is healing and has been recognised for many thousands of years by ancient Egyptian, Indian, Greek, Roman and Chinese cultures. The direct mechanical effect of rhythmically applied manual pressure improves blood circulation to muscles and soft tissue, and enhances the action of the surrounding immune tissue and lymphatics (the drainage channels for lymph fluid of the immune system). Gentle stroking of the skin triggers the release of endorphins, the body's natural pain killers related to opium and morphine. The stimulation of endorphins leads to a sense of peace and well being as well as pain relief. Massage also relieves stress, which is well known to influence other diseases.

MASSAGE IS HEALING.

Masseurs claim massage can improve arthritic joints. While massage can certainly decrease the tension and inflammation of the soft tissue surrounding a joint, thereby giving pain relief and increased mobility, it's doubtful whether it improves the actual joint due to the difficulty in massaging a bone. Massage also applies a gentle stretching action to the muscles and surrounding connective tissues that helps keep these tissues elastic. There are many different types of massage including Swedish massage, Japanese shiatsu, Indian ayurveda massage and Thai massage. Some other alternative therapies, such as aromatherapy, osteopathy and reflexology, incorporate massage as part of their treatment. Massage shouldn't hurt; if it does, find another masseur.

REFLEXOLOGY

Foot massage originated in China about 5000 years ago and was also used in ancient Egypt. Reflexologists claim that pressure applied to reflex points on the feet, which correspond to areas on the body, leads to stimulation of natural healing powers—the auric field—in the affected area. This promotes well being by increasing circulation and specific bodily and muscular functions. Reflexologists believe the feet and hands are more sensitive than most of us realise. Just as we use our eyes to detect light and movement, we use our hands and feet to detect pressure and movement, to stretch and to work out weight distribution.

Reflexologists also believe that toxins and waste matter accumulate at the reflex points in the feet and that foot massage will break down these accumulations. The breakdown in accumulations leads to a free energy flow along zones within the body, removes emotional debris, opens blocked nerve pathways, and increases blood circulation to the affected area which improves removal of the toxins from the damaged areas. They also believe certain areas of the feet represent states of mind and that reflex pressure can help with emotional problems or stress-related conditions.

There is no scientific evidence that reflexology can improve arthritis or for that matter any other condition, but at a recent international reflexology symposium in China, it was claimed that reflexology helped to alleviate pain in up to 94 per cent of cases. There are over 7000 nerve endings in each foot, so it could be postulated that pressure and massage of these nerve endings can induce feelings of deep relaxation, which is helpful to anyone with an ailment.

IT IS CLAIMED THAT REFLEXOLOGY PROVIDES PAIN RELIEF IN UP TO 94 PER CENT OF PATIENTS.

CHIROPRACTIC

'Chiropractic' comes from the Greek word and is loosely translated as 'manipulation by hand'. Chiropractic was invented in 1895 by a Canadian, Daniel Palmer, who was soon ostracised by the medical fraternity and later jailed for practising medicine without a licence. Despite this, the therapy became popular with patients (although not with medical doctors) and is now probably the most widely practised alternative therapy in the Western world. In the United States there are 55,000 registered chiropractic practitioners alone and it is the third largest health care profession in that country.

CHIROPRACTIC IS PROBABLY THE MOST WIDELY PRACTISED COMPLEMENTARY THERAPY IN THE WESTERN WORLD.

Chiropractic is based on the premise that the spine and spinal cord is the major pathway to total body health as it is the main communicating highway between the brain and the rest of the body. Any malalignment of the spinal column leads to the rest of the body becoming unhealthy— manipulation of the spine into proper position is at the heart of chiropractic practice, thereby allowing the body's natural healing processes to work in harmony. Keeping an arthritic joint aligned correctly minimises the stresses on it and an unstressed joint is much healthier. Chiropractic can be helpful for arthritis of the spine, hips, knees and shoulders.

Studies (published in reputable medical journals such as the *British Medical Journal*) have confirmed that chiropractic therapy for lumbar spine problems is not only beneficial but is also a relatively cheap way of treating these disorders.

Chiropractors use varying degrees of manipulative pressure depending on the state of the spine and the disease being treated—this is the main distinction between different schools and techniques of chiropractic. There are the more traditional forms where the chiropractor uses a short, rapid thrust to manipulate the spine. There are also forms that use low force techniques of gentle spine mobilisation. For very young children and the frail, chiropractors use an activator, a rubber-tipped instrument which is designed to deliver a very small thrust. If the joint is arthritic it is better to go gently and manipulate over several sessions rather than going for one big jolt and a well-trained chiropractor should take this into account.

OSTEOPATHY

The major difference between osteopathy and chiropractic is that osteopaths also use soft tissue therapy to relax muscles and improve joint mobility and function.

The word 'osteopathy' is another derivative from ancient Greek meaning 'disease of the bone'. Developed in North America during the Civil War by Dr Andrew Still, it's well accepted and widely practised in the west. Most of its popularity is based on its success in treating lower back complaints (although, during the flu epidemic of 1919, the survival rates in osteopathic hospitals in the United States far outstripped those in conventional hospitals).

OSTEOPATHY ALSO LOOKS AT LIFESTYLE, EMOTIONS AND DIET WHEN TREATING DISEASE.

Osteopathy is a holistic approach and takes into account lifestyle, emotions and diet in the treatment of disease. Osteopaths believe the best healing system available is the body's immune system and stimulation of this system is the best way to help a disease.

Osteopaths improve the mobility of arthritic joints and soft tissue using touch, manipulation, deep tactile pressure, stretching, massage, rhythmic passive joint mobilisation and rapid high-velocity thrust mobilisation of joints. He or she will more likely use gentle release techniques if you're frail. Osteopaths apply precise amounts of force to the body to promote movement of the body's fluids, to eliminate abnormal function in the motion of body tissues and to release compressed bones and joints. The areas being treated also need proper positioning to help the body's ability to regain normal tissue function.

NATUROPATHY

Naturopathic medicine began in the 19th century and was attractive to people reacting against the disease, dirt and grime of the Industrial Revolution, as well as often misguided medical practices. The European founders of naturopathy advocated a return to nature—exposure to sunlight, fresh air and water, hot springs and mineral spas to cure ills. From this, naturopathy evolved as a rival to Western medicine until the development of antibiotics and other modern medical treatments.

Much of Western medicine has its origins in naturopathy. Most of what we now call preventive medicine was taught by naturopaths for the whole of the 20th century. Common sense dictates that excessive lifestyles lead to medical problems and a healthy diet is crucial to a healthy life. Naturopathy is about more than just a healthy diet and has a holistic orientation.

Naturopaths believe the body has an inherent 'life force' that has the ability to establish, maintain and restore health. Their role is to facilitate and improve this life force, while at the same time removing any barriers to health and recovery by creating a healthy internal and external environment. They believe the equilibrium of the body is disturbed by an unhealthy lifestyle and so do not just treat the person's symptoms but try to get to the bottom of the problem. This is also the basis of preventive medicine.

A healthy diet is combined with non-invasive therapies such as herbal remedies, posture and breathing exercises, hydrotherapy, massage and osteopathy to try to bring relief. Unless the herbs are toxic or interact with other more traditional medicines that you've been prescribed, this would not be damaging. Some naturopaths also combine therapies and may use chiropractic, osteopathy, homeopathy and psychological counselling.

It is difficult to recommend one herbal treatment over another, as opinions vary. Each year several 'new' naturopathic cures for arthritis hit the market, most of which are aggressively promoted by their manufacturers for commercial profit. Some recent examples are ginger extract (ginger works for arthritis because it's full of salicylic acid which is aspirin); celery extract (used in Chinese herbal medicine); glucosamine for osteoarthritis which stimulates the formation of cartilage in damaged joints and has a weak anti-inflammatory action; New Zealand green-tipped muscle extract (which has had some success) and copper salves or bracelets.

MAKE SURE HERBAL REMEDIES WILL NOT ADVERSELY INTERACT WITH ANY OTHER MEDICATION YOU MAY BE TAKING.

Some of the remedies recommended by naturopaths for osteoarthritis include eating less refined foods, saturated animal fats and sugar, and eating more cereals, fresh fruit, and vegetables. Herbal remedies include juniper, feverfew, willow, aloe gel, wintergreen, alfalfa, chamomile, dandelion, peppermint tea and devil's claw. For rheumatoid arthritis you may be recommended a similar diet as for osteoarthritis, or an exclusion diet as naturopaths suspect food hypersensitivities aggravate rheumatoid arthritis. Fish oils, evening primrose oil, turmeric, skullcap and soy beans have anti-inflammatory properties.

Other herbals used in rheumatoid arthritis include burdock, gentian, sarsaparilla, wild yam, hops and nettle teas. Naturopaths believe that a copper deficiency is a factor in rheumatoid arthritis and so recommend the use of copper. For psoriatic arthritis, linseed oil both internally and rubbed over the inflamed joint may be recommended (although the smell might be off-putting).

For gout, naturopaths may recommend avoiding liver, kidneys, anchovies, meat extracts, yeasts and citric juices. Herbs they may recommend are celery, globe artichoke, pennyroyal oil, dandelion tea, apple cider poultices to the joint. They will also suggest you drink lots of fluids.

DIET THERAPY
Some specific diets are said to improve some arthritic conditions. While many Western medical practioners generally promote a well-balanced, conventional diet and are sceptical of restrictive and unusual diets, there

could still be some value in certain diets. For example, it took Western medicine considerably longer than natural therapists to recognise the adverse affects of cholesterol on the heart.

However I have found that most of my patients stop following these diets without any prompting from me because they are often unpalatable or bland. I have enough trouble trying to convince my cardiac patients to stay on a long-term low cholesterol diet because it's 'boring'. If you like the taste and palate of the diet and it's balanced, there is no reason not to use it, and if it helps your arthritis at the same time it's a bonus. If certain vitamins are missing in a diet you may need to add a vitamin supplement.

SPECIFIC DIETS SHOULD GIVE YOU ENOUGH
NUTRIENTS, VITAMINS AND MINERALS.

Some diets that apparently help arthritis include:

▶ the macrobiotic diet which recommends particular foods depending on their Chinese *yin* and *yang* properties
▶ the vegan diet for rheumatoid arthritis — this is vegetarianism which also excludes eggs, dairy products and honey
▶ the detoxification diet using fruits, raw vegetables and yoghurt to eliminate toxins from the body
▶ the elimination diet which avoids food sensitivities in rheumatoid arthritis
▶ the fish oil diet — fish oils are thought to work by reducing the inflammation in the joint.

HERBAL MEDICINE

Over 80 per cent of the world's people rely on herbs for health. Western medicine is still discovering 'new' herbal remedies, but at least 40 per cent of the currently available pharmaceuticals have a herbal origin. Probably the two most common herbal remedies used in Western medicine are digoxin (a cardiac drug), which is naturally found in foxglove, and strong pain killers such as morphine, which is derived from the opium poppy and is grown commercially (rather than illegally) in India and Tasmania.

Herbal medicine dates back to ancient times. There is evidence on clay tablets of the use of herbal medicine in the Sumerian civilisation in

Mesopotamia dating back to 4000 BC. Herbal medicine reached its peak in Western society between the 16th and 18th centuries and was especially popularised with the advent of printing, allowing the spread of information to anyone who could read. When the pilgrims first arrived in America they brought with them their own medicinal herbs to grow. From the Native Americans, and through trial and error, herbalists learned which plants in America could be used medicinally. But with the growth of science in the 18th century, and the medical profession's fascination and obsession with pharmaceutical chemistry, herbal medicine became less popular.

Herbalists believe disease is a disruption of the body's harmony and remedies given restore the body's harmony. They also believe the effect of herbs is not just from one chemical within a plant, but from the many chemicals acting in synergy. For example, the salicylic acid in meadowsweet is beneficial in rheumatic diseases but because meadowsweet also contains tannins, which protect the stomach lining, it can be used safely if you have a stomach disorder such as an ulcer.

HERBALISTS MAY RECOMMEND AN INFUSION OF DETOXIFYING HERBS AS A TREATMENT FOR ARTHRITIS.

You can use treatments externally or internally. You can apply cabbage leaves as a poultice to an arthritic joint every two to four hours to help settle the swelling and pain. The herbalist will soak cabbage leaves in hot water, wring them out and wrap them around the joint with cotton bandages. Internal treatments for arthritis may include tinctures or infusions of detoxifying herbs, such as celery seeds, to improve elimination of wastes from the body, and bitter herbs, such as devil's claw, to improve digestion.

A herbalist's skill in knowing the actions of different herbs on different organs in the body is similar to a Western medical doctor's knowledge of drugs. The acceptance of herbal therapy is growing in the Western world, particularly when the medicinal claims for herbs are supported by research and fact. In Europe and Australia, governments require a herbal remedy to be backed by scientific evidence before they are allowed to be marketed with medicinal claims. This motivates herbal manufacturing companies to research their products which has led to more research on herbal medicines.

CHINESE HERBAL MEDICINE

The first document relating to Chinese medicine, *Nei Jing* (*The Yellow Emperor's Classic of Internal Medicine*), dates back over 2000 years and relates to the ancient Chinese Taoist philosophy of moderation, balance and harmony. The first document relating to herbal treatments is from the 3rd century AD. According to Chinese legend, Shen Nung, the originator of Chinese agriculture, tested hundreds of different plants one by one, to discover their nutritional and medicinal properties. Many turned out to be poisonous.

The key principles of Chinese medicine relate to the three main Chinese beliefs of holism (the body as an interrelated whole), *yin* and *yang* and the five elements. Holism means that a person's arthritis doesn't just affect the joint but also other parts of the body. Running through the body are meridians of life energy, *qi*, which nourish the body's organs. If *qi* is disturbed, the disturbance is transmitted to the rest of the body. *Yin* and *yang* are the opposing but complementary forces of nature such as male/female, sun/moon and overcast/sunshine present in the body. The *yin* and *yang* are continually changing into their opposites such as day turns into night—each defines the other (without night you would not know what day was). *Yin* at one end of the spectrum is necessary for *yang* to exist at the other end and vice versa. *Yin* and *yang* are polar but unified. When the balance of *yin* and *yang* are disturbed, disease or emotional problems follow. The five elements of the universe—fire, earth, metal, water and wood—exist in the organs of the body. The elements support or inhibit each other (water dowses fire, fire melts metal) and this occurs in the body also, for example the kidneys (water) control the heart (fire) and the heart controls the lungs (metal).

CHINESE HERBAL REMEDIES BALANCE THE BODY'S FORCES, SO THAT HARMONY RESULTS.

Herbal remedies in Chinese medicine are used to re-balance these forces in the body. Herbs are classified by the quality of their five elements according to taste—sweet, sour, bitter, pungent and salty. The *yin* and *yang* qualities of hot and cold are also linked to specific actions of herbs. For example, skullcap (*huang quin*) is a bitter, cold herb used to lower fever. Each herb works in specific organs and meridians and is usually prescribed in a formula of up to 10 or more herbs. Each herb has a different role and its presence in the formula depends on the person's age, constitution, and pattern of disharmony.

Pokeberries (*shang-lu*) are a Chinese remedy for the aches and pains of arthritis which you can use as a tincture. To dissolve toxic build-ups of inflammatory chemicals in the joints, you can make a herbal tea with *fo-ti-tieng* roots. It's regarded as a good remedy for bursitis, gout and arthritis. Ginseng root is classified as an anti-rheumatic and is more potent if processed into a compound tea. Celery (*han-ch'in*), as well as being a food, is also used as an anti-arthritic, for gout and neuralgia. Celery seeds are made into a strong tea, which is said to neutralise uric acids and other excess acids in the body. Celery is also used in traditional Japanese medicine for arthritis relief. Western medicine has found the high levels of organic sodium in celery help keep calcium in solution within the blood so it can be eliminated from the body. In chronic inflammation calcium is deposited in the inflamed tissues such as tendons and capsules of joints—celery reduces the inflammation.

Queen of the meadow (*lan-ts'ao*) is used for back pain due to strains. You can drink it as a tea but a compound formula of *lan-ts'ao* with burdock (*wu-shih*), *shang-lu* and flaxseed (*shih-ma*) gives rapid relief of gout and other forms of arthritis. Although you can buy Chinese herbs over the counter, they are more effective if you consult a Chinese herbalist for an individual prescription.

Pastes, poultices, creams, ointments, lotions or liniments of herbs can also give some relief. Tiger balm is used for minor arthritic aches and pains. Cajeput oil, which is distilled from the cajeput tree leaves, smells like a combination of camphor and eucalyptus and is rubbed on inflamed joints. For quick relief of back pain and sciatica, use hops (*hu-ts'ao*) in a warm to hot poultice. Mugwort (*ai-hao*) leaves are steamed and used as a poultice for pain relief. Rosemary (*mi-tieh-hsiang*) was brought to China from Rome during the Wei dynasty—mix with juniper oil and use as a liniment for relief of back ache. To reduce joint inflammation and arthritic pain use peanut oil (*hua-shen-yu*) as a warm massaging oil. It is a slow relief and needs continuous three-times-a-day application. Camphor (*chang*) is mixed in small amounts with Chinese wine and used as a liniment for aches and pains.

ACUPUNCTURE

Acupuncture is at least 5000 years old. Stone needles have been found in Mongolia dating to this time and needles made of metal, such as gold and silver, date back 2000 years. Acupuncture is part of Chinese traditional medicine and incorporates the concepts of *qi*, *yin* and *yang* and meridians of energy. There are 12 meridians running up and down the body in pairs, six on either side of the body. They are also grouped in six *yin* of solid organs and six *yang* of hollow organs such as the stomach. There are also two controlling meridians, the conception and governing meridians. *Qi* is required to circulate evenly throughout the body, otherwise disease will occur. There are up to 365 acupuncture points along each meridian at which point *qi* is concentrated and can enter and leave the body. By introducing needles at these acupuncture points it's possible to stimulate or suppress the flow of *qi* and influence the disease. To stay healthy, your *qi* needs to circulate evenly throughout your body.

ACUPUNCTURE CONTROLS PAIN IN ARTHRITIC CONDITIONS AND MAY SUPPRESS THE DISEASE.

Western researchers have not been able to measure the *qi* energy. Some theories suppose the energy transfer is a form of transmission of neurochemical messages to the brain. Other theories suggest that acupuncture transfers messages to the brain via pressure rather than through electrical/nerve pathway messages. Whatever the mechanism, acupuncture is successful, especially to control pain in arthritic conditions. It may also suppress arthritis disease. There is little chance of any damage being induced by acupuncture and the World Health Organization currently lists 43 diseases and conditions that can be treated with it.

AYURVEDA

Ayuverda is the major holistic traditional healing therapy of India and uses a combination of purifying techniques, diet, yoga, massage, herbal remedies and breathing exercises to improve physical, mental, emotional and spiritual health. The word 'ayurveda' comes from the Sanskrit meaning 'science of life' (*ayu* = life, *veda* = knowledge) and has been used in India for at least 2500 years. Like traditional Chinese medicine, it maintains a strong connection between mind and the body and there is no separation of philosophy and medicine.

When the British Raj controlled India, there was a concerted attempt to stamp out ayurveda. After Indian independence in 1947, the practice was revitalised and the government encouraged control of standards. Ayurveda is now growing in popularity throughout the rest of the world.

Ayurveda philosophy teaches there are three *doshas*, or vital energies, that influence human beings and are continually fluctuating in their proportions in nature. Each of the *doshas* is made up of a combination of two of the five elements of the universe: ether, air, fire, water and earth, and these combinations create various physiological functions within the body. *Vata dosha* is formed from air and ether and controls movement, nerve impulses, circulation, respiration and elimination. *Pitta dosha* is formed from water and fire and controls body metabolism and conversion of foods into energy. *Kapha dosha* is formed from earth and water and controls growth, cohesion and protection for the body.

The levels of *doshas* in the body are influenced by the external environment's *doshas*, the time of day, different foods eaten, the season, stress levels and emotional state. Imbalances in the *doshas* disrupt the flow of life energy, *prana*, that enters the body via food and breath and interfere with digestive fire, *agni*, which processes food and experiences. If *agni* is low, toxic substances called *ama* are produced that cause illnesses. Ayurveda places great emphasis on diet and detoxification in preventing and treating illnesses. Herbal remedies, yoga, meditation and massage are all thought to balance the *doshas* and improve the level of *prana*.

AYURVEDA STRESSES THE IMPORTANCE OF DIET AND DETOXIFICATION IN PREVENTING AND TREATING ILLNESSES.

We all have different proportions of *doshas* in our body, so treatment regimes for a particular ailment vary depending on the uniqueness of the combinations of *doshas*. When any of the *doshas* over-accumulate, ayurveda suggests specific lifestyle and nutritional guidelines to help the individual reduce the excess. You may also be recommended herbal supplements to speed up the the healing process and the primary method of returning the *doshas* to equilibrium is through diet.

Substantial research has been done on ayurveda at the Government Medical College, Jammu, India. A study specifically for rheumatoid arthritis showed 122 out of 175 people with this disease improved when they were treated with *boswellia serrata*, a common herb used in ayurveda. Other treatments have shown a decrease in the size of cancerous tumours in rats and reduced cholesterol and anxiety levels in people with heart disease.

HOMEOPATHY

The word 'homeopathy' loosely translates from the ancient Greek meaning 'same suffering'. The premise of homeopathy is that small doses of a substance, which in large doses is poisonous to the body, will cure symptoms of the poisonous condition. This principle dates back to the time of Hippocrates in the 5th century BC, and was rediscovered by a German doctor, Samuel Hahnemann in 1810. He summarised homeopathy with the Latin phrase *similia similibus curentur*, which means 'let likes cure likes'. As well as using dilutions of toxins, homeopaths also take into account your constitutional classification (personality and habit traits).

The homeopathic treatment given to you will vary depending on your symptoms and constitution—different people with the same disease and symptoms will not necessarily be treated with the same homeopathic dilute toxins. Homeopathic treatment is accepted especially in Europe, Australia and India, and is becoming increasingly popular in the United States.

HOMEOPATHY WORKS ON THE PREMISE THAT LIKE CURES LIKE, SO SMALL DOSES OF WHAT AILS YOU MAY BE GIVEN TO COUNTER THE SYMPTOMS OF YOUR CONDITION.

There is now a scientific explanation of homeopathy based on electron orbit and electron energy changes in atoms (patented by a French company listed on the Australian Stock Exchange, Medicine Quantale). The basic theory is that the introduction of a homeopathic toxin will induce structural electron changes in the atom, which then leads to changes in the energy levels of the atom. This in turn leads to a relief of symptoms and a cure. The electron changes, then becomes permanently embedded in the structure of the atom, resulting in immune protection and stimulation.

Homeopathic doses of a toxin are extremely dilute so the toxin doesn't damage your body when you take it. It's said that a 12c homeopathic dilution is the equivalent to a pinch of salt in the ocean. Some examples are: dilutions of spring grass pollens as a treatment for hayfever and asthma, and belladonna as a treatment for scarlet fever (belladonna poisoning symptoms are similar to scarlet fever). Gout can be treated by ledum 6c, colchicum 6c, arnica 6c, urtica 6c or pulsatilla 6c depending on your main symptoms. Ankylosing spondylosis (see Chapter 12) can respond to either arnica 6c or rhus tox 6c.

Homeopathic treatment in rheumatoid arthritis has been proven to be as effective as salicylic acid for symptom relief. Research at the Glasgow Homoeopathic Hospital in 1986 found that homeopathic treatment for rheumatoid arthritis is as effective as the disease-modifying drugs currently used by Western medicine—and that the homeopathic treatment was much safer to use.

ENVIRONMENTAL MEDICINE

Environmental medicine is based on the idea that many chronic disorders, including inflammatory arthritis, are caused by environmental exposure to foods, pesticides, pollen, dust, exhaust fumes and other pollutants. Environmental therapists claim that drinking unfiltered tap water and eating a typical Western diet exposes you to at least 100 environmental synthetic toxins, including pesticides, herbicides, residues of drugs fed to animals before slaughter and preservatives in processed food. These environmental toxins don't necessarily induce full-blown allergic reactions with itching, rashes and swelling, but can lead to other diseases and intolerances.

Environmental therapists believe that if you have concurrent infections or a diet deficient in antioxidant vitamins and minerals you are especially sensitive to environmental illness. This will also make you prone to inflammatory reactions and alterations in your brain chemistry (induced by environmental toxins), which alter your mood and sap vitality. Therapists try to identify the causative toxins to help you avoid them. They also try to improve your diet with oral and intravenous vitamins and may also try to desensitise your immune system to particular toxins and retrain it to eliminate allergies. You may also be recommended detoxification to remove metals and chemicals from your body. There is no scientific evidence to prove that arthritis is caused by exposure to environmental toxins.

HYPNOTHERAPY

'Hypnotism' is the Greek word for 'sleep'. Not used as a direct cure for arthritis, it can help you relax, become less stressed and may even give you some pain relief (probably through muscle relaxation). If you have arthritis you have to deal with lifestyle changes, financial strains and possible relationship changes, as well as the disease itself. Any technique that reduces stress levels will be of benefit as you'll be able to cope better with the problems induced by your arthritis. This in itself will increase your pain relief, as stress makes you more susceptible to pain.

Hypnotism goes back to ancient Egyptian and Greek cultures where healing trances were induced for medical conditions. African and South American cultures also use hypnotic trances as part of their healing medicine. Hypnotism as it is known today is a result of work done by an Austrian doctor, Franz Mesmer, who was later branded a charlatan for his work. He believed illness was due to an imbalance in the body's magnetic field and insisted he could restore the imbalance by transferring magnetic forces from his own body to the patient's, by waving iron bars and magnets over the patient's heads and uttering soothing words at the same time to induce a trance. During the late 1800s hypnotism started to become more recognised by the medical community with 'schools' of hypnotism being set up in France. In the 1960s hypnotherapy took on its modern form and use when used in conjunction with psychotherapy in the United States.

Hypnotherapists claim that 90 per cent of people can be hypnotised. This happens when the conscious state is bypassed and the subconscious is made more receptive to suggestion. Hypnotherapy relies on the induction of a trance-like state to reach the subconscious state of mind, the level over which you usually have no control. Once the subconscious is open to suggestion the hypnotherapist can promote a new way of dealing with pain. If you're someone who is willing to be hypnotised, you can have minor surgery while you're in this altered conscious state.

While there seems to be little doubt that hypnotherapy provides a lasting benefit to many who try it, no one knows why. There has been speculation that hypnotic trances induce the release of the natural narcotics, endorphins, which results in decreased pain sensitivity. Another theory suggests that hypnosis acts through the subconscious part of the mind that controls involuntary actions such as breathing, hunger, heart rate, blood pressure and reactions to pain. Hypnosis allows you to gain some control over these functions.

FELDENKRAIS TECHNIQUE
A form of physical re-education of the body, the technique was developed in Israel during the 1950s by Russian-born atomic physicist, Moshe Feldenkrais. The Feldenkrais technique is particularly practised in Israel, the United States, Europe and Australia.

The method is not a treatment or cure but can be a supportive therapy for situations in which improved movement patterns can help you recover from illness or injury. Practitioners believe that habitual postures and movements represent disruptions in the nervous system and Feldenkrais techniques improve the ease of movement with minimum effort and maximum efficiency. This will enhance body awareness, flexibility, coordination, and range of joint movement. It will also give you a greater sense of well being. The technique aims to improve physical and mental well being by reprogramming movement patterns. To do this the therapist will help you develop body awareness and increase your joint mobility. Originally developed for patients with neurological disorders, such as cerebral palsy, it has also been successful in treating back complaints, including arthritis of the spine.

Poor posture will aggravate any arthritic condition so if you can be taught to recognise your own poor posture and how to improve it, then you will find relief from pain.

POOR POSTURE AGGRAVATES ARTHRITIS. FELDENKRAIS CAN HELP YOU RECOGNISE POOR POSTURE AND IMPROVE IT.

ALEXANDER TECHNIQUE

This technique is a body orientation therapy that helps to improve posture and lead to fewer stresses on arthritic joints. In the late 1890s, an Australian actor, Frederick Alexander, wanted to improve his speech delivery. He watched himself in the mirror, noting muscle tension, and taught himself to release these restrictive muscle actions. Alexander believed that habitual poor posture influences the way the body and mind function and that we need to relearn basic body postures to be able to function in a healthy way. The technique teaches you to become aware of patterns of misuse in your movements and learn basic body alignment. In this respect the background theory of the Alexander technique is similar to the Feldenkrais technique although the actual physical therapy is different. Musicians have used the technique to help them hold their instruments in the least stressful way, thus improving their playing.

The Alexander technique is generally well accepted by the traditional medical fraternity as a therapy for muscle and joint problems. It's especially helpful for painful back problems and can improve joint mobility, strength and decrease pain. It attempts to relieve musculoskeletal problems by discouraging habitual, counterproductive muscular reactions and allowing efficient natural reflexes to take over.

THE ALEXANDER TECHNIQUE CAN HELP RELIEVE BACK PAIN AND IMPROVE JOINT MOBILITY.

MAGNETIC THERAPY

Magnetic therapy was used in ancient China and Egypt and it's claimed that Cleopatra wore a magnet on her head to maintain her beauty. Magnet therapy was introduced into modern society by Dr Franz Mesmer at the same time he was experimenting with hypnotherapy. Mesmer waved metal wands over people's heads trying to improve their 'animal magnetism', a universal force he claimed flowed through everyone's body. Complementary practitioners believe weak magnetic fields set up by ordinary magnets can influence the body's cells and their intrinsic electrical currents to promote healing. The theory is the iron molecules in haemoglobin in red blood cells respond to magnetism leading to improved blood flow, oxygen supply, metabolism, and helps eliminate wastes from the magnetised area.

Current medical opinion in the United States and the United Kingdom accepts magnetic therapy as successful but only in high dose magnetic fields, as used for bone growth stimulation in treatment of fractures, wound healing and thrombosis, but doesn't accept the value of low dose magnetic fields to be therapeutic (despite these therapies being popular in Eastern Europe and Japan). Typically, for pain relief, a magnet is strapped to an arthritic joint with the magnet strength being about 500 gauss, which is about five to 10 times the strength of a typical fridge door magnet. It can be used for as little as three minutes or all day and can be used long-term for any recurrences that occur.

Magnetic therapy is totally unsuitable if you have a cardiac pacemaker or cardiac defibrillator, because the magnetic fields could induce malfunctioning of these machines. Also do not use magnetic therapy if you're pregnant.

CRYSTAL THERAPY

Crystals, especially quartz, topaz, rose quartz, amethyst and garnet, are thought to be able store and discharge healing 'life energy'. The crystal can be rubbed on the body, worn on the body, placed in a room that you're in or placed over acupuncture points or chakra points (centres of life energy used in yoga) of the body. Specific crystals that are thought to help arthritic conditions are carnelian, chysocolla, copper and sulphur crystals. There is no scientific evidence to support the claims of crystal therapists but shamanistic cultures throughout the world have used crystals for their magical and therapeutic effects.

CHAPTER | 4

LIFESTYLE

Exercise

Diet

Attitudes

Y our lifestyle plays a critical part in your health and well being. The three major aspects of a healthy way of life are exercise, diet and attitude.

EXERCISE

No matter which treatment option you decide to undertake, either Western medicine, complementary therapies or a combination of both, there is no more essential therapy than regular exercise. It doesn't have to be organised—staying active can be incorporated into your daily routine around the house or at work.

The aim of exercise in arthritis is not to bust your gut but to maintain the mobility and flexibility of your joints by moving them through a large but painless range. A joint that's not moved through its full range of movement regularly will stiffen up and eventually form a *contracture*. A contracture of a joint is a deformity as a result of scarring within the joint, limiting its movement. If the joint can't travel its full range, your flexibility is lost and mobility restricted.

Joints that aren't exercised also suffer from associated muscle wasting. Muscles need constant use to maintain their viability and if the joint isn't powered properly, the muscles will become less flexible. When astronauts return from a prolonged space visit, they have lost large amounts of muscle mass through weightlessness because they have been unable to walk or stand. Even if your arthritis is established, maintaining muscle mass by exercising helps to preserve joint function. The earlier you start an exercise regime, the less likely the risk of contractures, deformities and muscle wasting.

REGULAR EXERCISE BASED ON MOBILITY, FLEXIBILITY AND STRETCHING WILL HELP YOU MAINTAIN MUSCLE MASS AND KEEP THE JOINT FUNCTIONING.

Any exercise regime you do should not end in pain. A 'no pain, no gain' attitude will only lead to more problems with the joint—usually further damage. Exercise needs to be gentle and comfortable without causing increased physical stresses. It's better to use larger joints to perform an action rather than smaller ones as they cope better with physical stresses. Small joints are best used for fine motor control activities. For example, you could carry a bag on your shoulder rather than in your hand.

Base your exercise regimes around mobility, flexibility, stretching and relaxation. Before you start any activity, plan tasks so you don't stress a joint. If you're doing exercise classes as part of your exercise regime, it's OK to omit some exercises if you're getting tired or are starting to ache. Do the ones that you're comfortable with and rest if you need to. Introduce new exercises gradually and if repetitions are part of the regime, increase the numbers as your body develops endurance.

Of course, if you are in the middle of an acute arthritic flare-up, such as a gouty attack, exercise is the last thing you should do. Rest is a much better option during acute flare-ups until you are back to your normal state.

DON'T EXERCISE IF YOU HAVE AN ACUTE FLARE-UP OF ARTHRITIS SYMPTOMS.

Low impact exercise

If your arthritis affects hips, knees, feet and lower spine, you'll benefit most from low impact exercise. Swimming and water aerobics don't place any stresses on weight bearing joints and most people find them beneficial. One advantage of water-based exercise programs is that the buoyancy of water can help increase the range of movement and the resistance of the water helps increase muscle strength. Water allows smooth execution of movements— jerky, rushing movements don't help arthritic joints. In water, movements may act as a pain reliever and relaxant. Water-based exercise is aerobic, so it also improves heart fitness. Some pools have exercise classes for arthritis sufferers. Try to find a pool with ramp access or a hoist if you have a mobility problem.

IF ARTHRITIS IS AFFECTING YOUR HIPS, KNEES OR LOWER SPINE, SWIMMING AND WATER AEROBICS CAN PROVIDE GREAT RELIEF. THIS WILL ALSO HELP TO INCREASE THE STRENGTH OF YOUR MUSCLES.

Bicycle riding and stationary exercise bike riding are also aerobic and don't put weight bearing stress on your joints. Walking is also excellent but has its restrictions if you have major arthritic problems with your leg or spine joints—every time you step, your upper body weight is transferred through the lower spine, hips, knees and feet. About six times your body weight is absorbed by your knee joints, and if these joints are affected by arthritis, long walks are not going to be beneficial and will lead to further damage. You could either shorten your walks, or change your exercise regime altogether. If you decide to persist with walking, make sure your shoes are well cushioned or have orthotic inserts to minimise the abnormal forces acting on your joints. Consider two short walks instead of one long one and play only 9 holes of golf instead of 18.

Other forms of exercise

Passive movement exercise forms will also benefit you. Yoga, tai chi and some forms of dance all improve joint flexibility and motion without putting undue stresses on the joints. Let your teacher know that you have arthritis before you begin, as some of the exercises may need to be modified or left out. Some people recommend bouncer trampolines as an exercise for arthritis, but they may not minimise impact on joints. It's also easy to twist a joint on landing, which will damage even a normal joint.

Diversity in movement is important in any exercise regime you do. Repetitive movements are not healthy for normal joints unless the ergonomic situation is perfect. Keyboarders often develop repetitive strain injuries and tenosynovitis because the postures and positions used for typing are not ideal. If you have arthritis of the hands and fingers, knitting or crocheting as exercise for the hands will aggravate your arthritis because of the dynamics and repetitive movements. If you still want to do these activities, do them for short periods, preferably for less than 20 minutes at one time.

The most effective exercise regimes for arthritis stick to the principles of no pain, full range of joint movement, low repetition counts and low impact, and they aim to improve flexibility, mobility and muscle strength. If they overcome the boredom of repetitive exercise, it's a bonus. The following is a description of the range of movements that your joints should be able to make. If you have an arthritic joint slowly try to mobilise it through its full range of movement. If your joint already has well-established arthritis you may not be able to achieve full range—attempt the movements anyway as they will help retain the existing range.

Neck (Cervical spine)
1. Touch your chin onto your breastbone, then rotate your chin onto the tips of both your shoulders.
2. Put your right ear onto your right shoulder, then put your left ear onto your left shoulder.

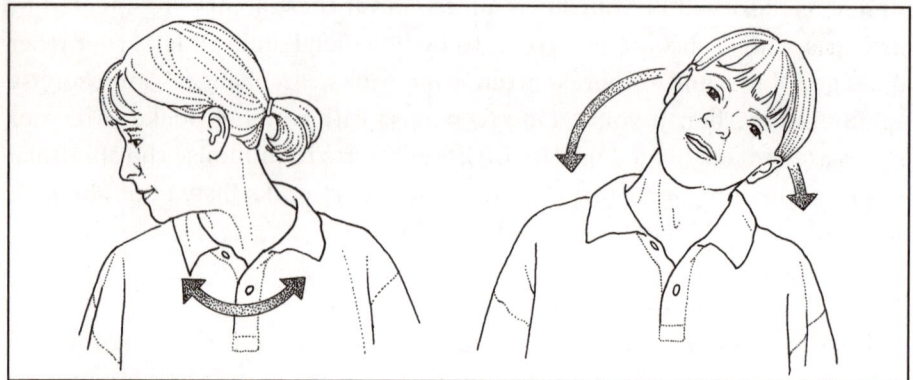

Mid-back (Thoracic spine)
1. With your chin on your breastbone hunch your shoulders forwards, as if you're going to roll yourself into a ball.
2. With your body standing at attention look to your left and right by rotating at the hips without twisting your neck.

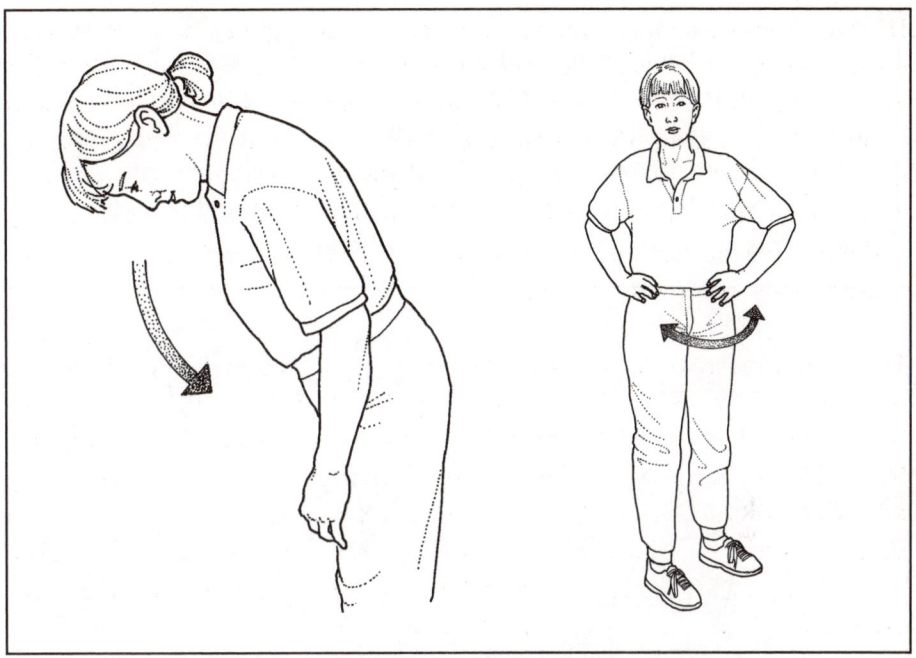

Lower back (Lumbar-sacral spine)

1. Bend over and try to touch your toes, keeping your knees straight.
2. Arch your back backwards as far as you can.
3. Bending sideways, run your right arm down the right thigh and calf, run the left arm down the left thigh and calf.

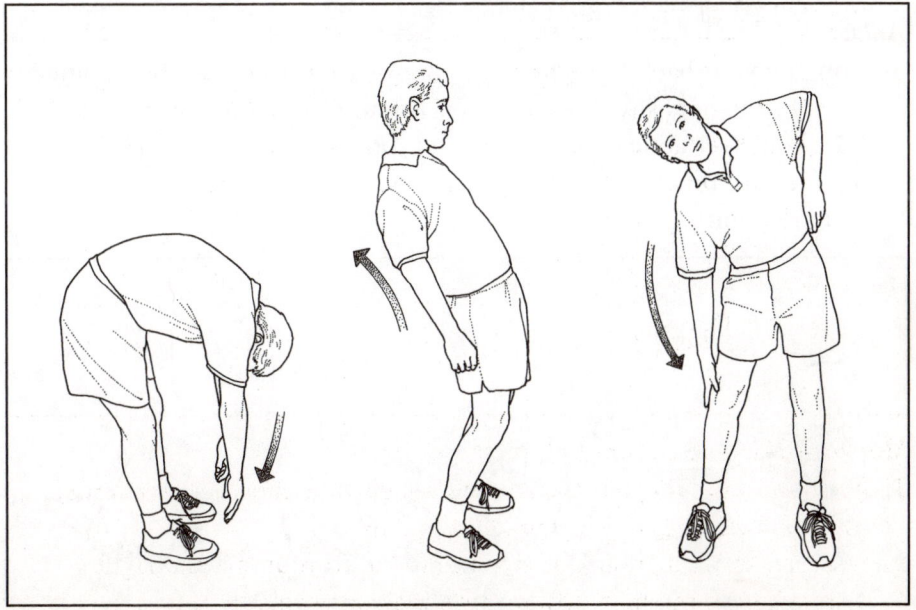

Hips

1. Lying on your back, bring both knees up to the chest.
2. Lying on your back spread your legs outwards as far as possible, keeping your legs straight and on the floor.
3. Sitting on a chair rotate your legs outwards and then inwards.
4. Lying on your left side, hold your right leg straight and push it backwards as far as you can. Repeat on the other side.

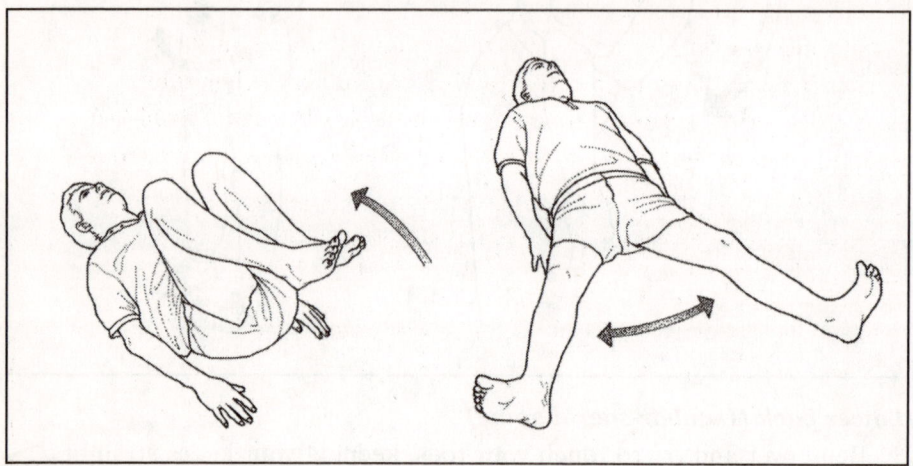

Knees

1. Straighten your knees as far as they will go and then bend them as far as they will go. Normally you can get about 120 degrees of movement.

Ankles

1. Lying on your back flex your feet towards your head and then point them in the opposite direction as if you were standing on tiptoes.
2. Have your feet about 30cm apart and rotate both ankles so that the big toes are touching. Then do the opposite movement so that the feet are pointing outwards.

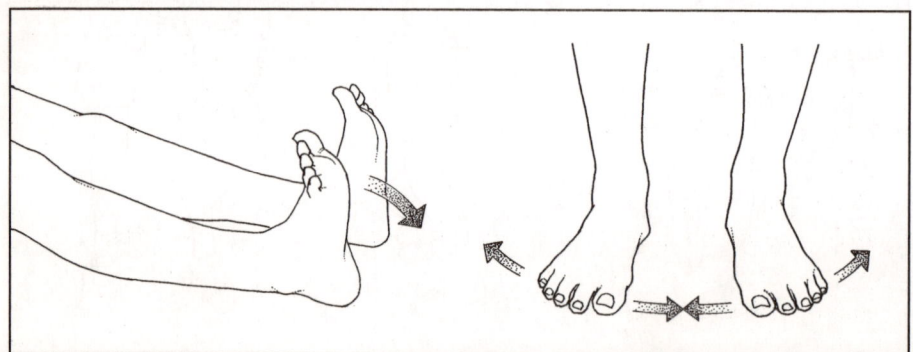

Toes

1. When sitting, bend all your toes towards your head and then imagine trying to pick up a golf ball by gripping it with your toes to the sole of the foot. Spread your toes inwards and outwards.

Shoulders

1. Holding your arm straight, extend it sideways and lift to touch your ear. Repeat other side
2. Holding your arm straight, move it forwards and upwards so that it lies against the corresponding ear. Repeat other side.
3. With the arm against your side and the elbow bent in a fixed 90° angle, rotate the arm outwards. Reach backwards and try to touch the bottom of your opposite shoulder blade. Repeat other side.

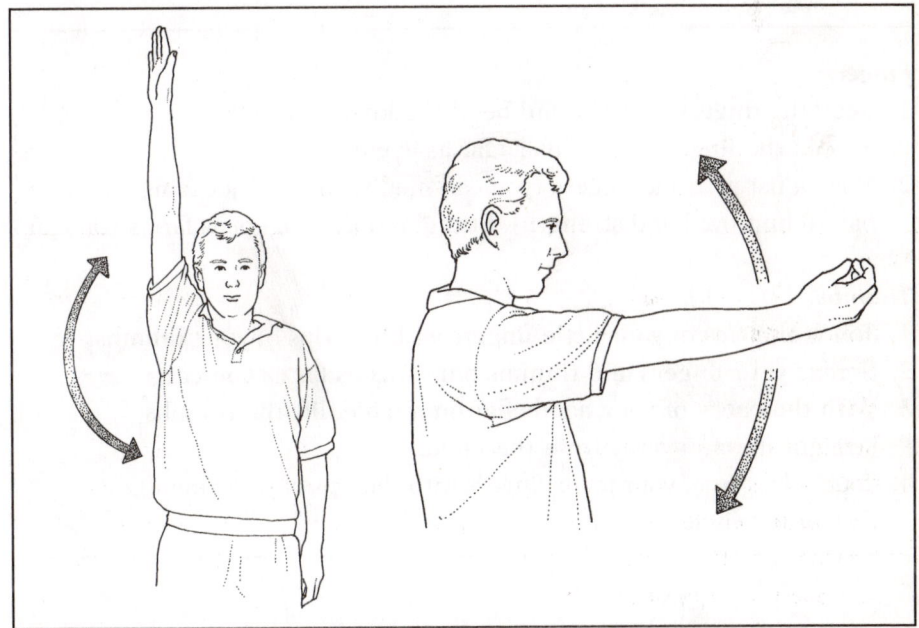

Elbows

1. Straighten the elbow as far as you can. Bend the elbow and touch your shoulder with your fingertips. Repeat other side.
2. Hold your arms straight out in front of you. Rotate your palms to face upwards and then downwards.

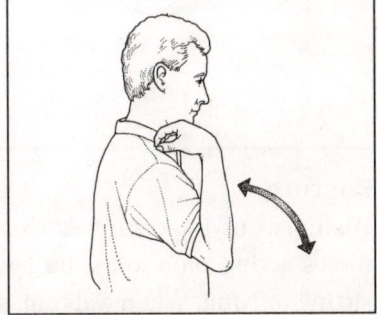

Wrists
1. Flex your hands backwards and forwards as far as you can.
2. Flex your hands from side to side.

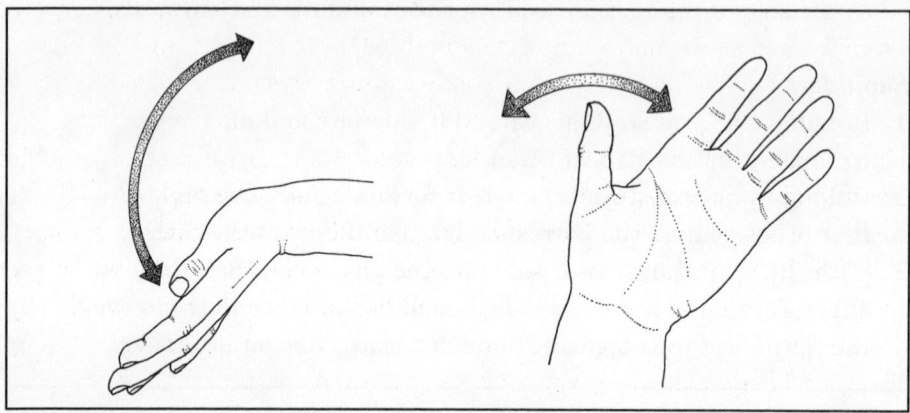

Fingers
1. Keep the fingers straight and bend the knuckles to 90°.
   Spread the fingers outwards as far as you can.
2. Make a fist with the fingers (you can modify this by squeezing a squash ball to improve hand strength). Straighten the fingers as far as you can.

Thumbs
1. Touch the tips of your little fingers with the tips of your thumbs.
2. Spread your fingers and thumbs outwards as far as you can.
3. With the backs of your hands flat on a table, lift the thumbs straight upwards away from the table.
4. Touch the tips of your index fingers with the tips of your thumbs and form a circle.

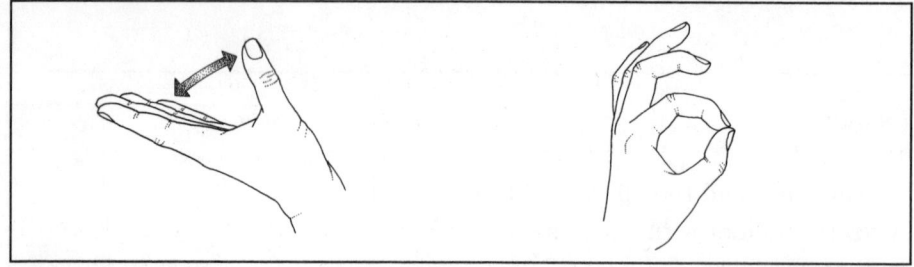

Posture
Posture is as important as exercise, as proper posture decreases abnormal forces acting on a joint. Be aware of your posture when standing, walking, sitting or lying. When walking, sitting or just standing, try to make sure your

back is straight, and your shoulders and chin are horizontal to the ground. Relax your shoulders, as a totally rigid posture is just as bad as a slouched or slumped one. Avoid sitting or standing for long periods. Take breaks every 20 to 30 minutes to alter your position and posture, and change positions as often as you can. If you're carrying something, such as a bag, make sure you swap sides frequently so that your posture doesn't become lop-sided.

Choosing good furniture will also help your posture. Work chairs should have good lower back support and armchairs need to be high backed (for neck support), firm seated and straight backed for better lumbar support. Bed selection is also critical for posture. Any mattress with a sag in the middle will tend to roll you into the middle of the bed, which won't help your arthritic spine. Mattresses recommended by the Chiropractic Society for optimal spinal posture are available from most retail bedding shops.

DIET

With the exception of gout (see Chapter 13), there is no scientific proof that a particular diet will improve or worsen an arthritic condition. But common sense tells us the benefits of a healthy balanced diet. If you're overweight, you'll increase your arthritic problems because your joints have to carry extra weight. Obese people have over four times the risk of developing knee osteoarthritis than people of average weight, and for every 5 kg of weight you gain, the risk of knee osteoarthritis increases by 35 per cent. If you already have knee osteoarthritis, losing weight can improve your symptoms of joint pain and slow progression of the disease. Pain in a joint is a good motivator for losing weight—even a weight loss of 5 to 10 kg will improve your quality of life.

IF YOU ARE OVERWEIGHT YOU WILL INCREASE YOUR ARTHRITIC PROBLEMS BECAUSE YOUR JOINTS HAVE TO CARRY EXTRA WEIGHT.

A weight-reducing diet means eating smaller amounts of food, especially if your activity level is decreased by arthritis. However it is important to eat the right sort of food. You still need to eat a balanced diet so you get all the essential nutrients. A balanced diet includes small amounts of processed sugars and fats, moderate amounts of lean meats for protein and unrestricted levels of cereals, carbohydrates and fruit and vegetables.

There are many diets that promise a cure for this or that disease, including arthritis, but not one of them appears to have stood the test of time. If you feel a diet may help you, try it, but if, after several weeks, your symptoms haven't improved, don't feel you have to persist with it.

ATTITUDES

The body and mind are closely intermeshed—your body won't be able to tolerate the degrees of change induced by arthritis without corresponding changes in your mind. Depression is the most common psychological reaction to limitations and changes of the body and results in a total lack of motivation—and you need to be motivated to cope with arthritis.

THE BODY AND THE MIND ARE CLOSELY INTERMESHED.
FEELINGS OF DEPRESSION ARE COMMON WHEN
ARTHRITIS TAKES A HOLD ON THE BODY.

Depression

Most people only need sensitive suggestions and prompting to overcome the problem of depression. This could come from your doctor, your physiotherapist, your herbalist or someone close to you. But you may become so depressed that it interferes with your ability to develop any coping strategies and need professional help. It's tempting to blame yourself or others for your arthritis as a defence mechanism. If you're depressed, psychiatrists and psychologists can help you understand these reactions, come to terms with your changing situation and help you to develop positive coping attitudes.

Fear

You may also find your diagnosis of arthritis frightening. You may be afraid of the consequences of the arthritis; of the treatments offered and the side effects of drugs; of falling because of unstable balance; of employment problems; of the discomfort of travelling; of not coping; and of overdoing things. The biggest fear could be ending up in a wheelchair. If you have an understanding of your arthritis it's easier to be positive about your life and not be afraid of the consequences. A great deal of fear comes from not knowing how things will turn out, so find out as much as you can about your condition and your fears are likely to diminish, your confidence will improve, your coping strategies will increase and you can adjust your thinking accordingly. Despite your arthritis, you will become more in control of what you want to do in your life. It may take a little while to overcome your fears, and it's natural to be nervous about some things, but don't let fear interfere in your life unnecessarily.

Anger

Expect to feel angry about arthritis. Anger is one of the emotions that you need to work through before you can deal with your future. You have every right to be angry at your arthritis so scream, shout and rage if that's the best way for you, but work through it quickly. Try not to get stuck in a rut about it because if you stay fixated by the anger you'll never achieve the more important things in your life. You won't be a pleasant person to be with if all you express are feelings of hostility, resentment and indignation. There's more to life than these negative emotions. Being involved in other things dissipates your anger as well as letting you get on with your life.

IF YOU CAN NO LONGER PARTICIPATE IN CERTAIN ACTIVITIES BECAUSE OF YOUR ARTHRITIS, SEEK OUT NEW IDEAS AND NEW ACTIVITIES.

Guilt

You might also feel guilt. For example, you might think that someone close to you will miss out on things because you're no longer able to join in some activities. You may have enjoyed ballroom dancing with your partner, an activity no longer possible because of your aches. This is a natural reaction but don't feel bad about yourself—you have other activities to offer. Guilt comes from negative self-images, of feelings that you're a 'bad' person. Just because you've developed arthritis doesn't mean you have suddenly become a 'bad' person. It doesn't make sense to feel guilty about arthritis.

Boredom

When you develop a disease that restricts what you want to do, you can get bored. First, recognise your capabilities. Drop the activities you can no longer do. Also don't go around thinking you can't do anything because of arthritis. Analyse the reasons for your boredom and then work out what you can do about it. Add other interests to your life and don't limit yourself to things you used to enjoy. Expand your horizons and change your preferences. Learn something new—learning is the quickest way to overcome boredom.

Stress

All your feelings about arthritis can make you stressed. Stress is a normal physiological response that makes the body maximise its efficiency. It helps you mobilise your strength physically and mentally to help you deal with and adapt to the different things that are occurring in your life. Most people think of stress as negative but stress can also be positive—in small amounts it helps you to handle your life in the best possible way. It's only when you become overwhelmed by too much stress that you can't cope and stress becomes a negative focus. Excess stress leads to nervousness, tension, anxiety and anger and some people are more vulnerable to this than others.

The way you cope with stress depends on your upbringing, your self-esteem, your beliefs about yourself and how you guide yourself in your thoughts and actions. The degree to which you feel in control of your life will determine your response to stress and your response will also be influenced by how you get along with people. Because everyone's combination of thoughts and behaviours are different, your coping mechanisms will be unique.

IF MANAGED WELL, STRESS HAS A POSITIVE EFFECT ON THE BODY.

Prolonged stress can be harmful. When your body is strong it can fight off most germs and diseases but prolonged stress puts such a strain on your body your defence mechanisms physically break down. This in turn makes you more vulnerable to the arthritis. When an animal is stressed, its reaction is either to fight or to run away. Humans have one big disadvantage compared with animals: their reaction to stress is usually mental rather than physical. Animals relieve their stress quickly, while humans scratch their heads thinking about the problem and achieve very little. Release of stress makes you feel better. If you don't relieve the stress, existing diseases get worse. You may even develop psychosomatic symptoms including abdominal pain, nausea and headaches.

If you're not dealing well with excess stress, ask your doctor or a psychologist for help. Both will have methods to help you reduce stress and get on with enjoying your life.

CHAPTER | 5

OSTEOARTHRITIS

O steoarthritis is the most common joint disease. It has a long history of afflicting humankind and has been found in the joints of Neanderthal skeletons. Palaeontologists have also found evidence of osteoarthritis in the ankle joints of dinosaurs.

Generally considered to be a non-inflammatory arthritis, new evidence suggests there's a localised inflammatory component within the joint itself. Unlike the recognised inflammatory arthritic diseases, it doesn't have consequences for other organs of the body and its effects remain restricted to the joint.

STATISTICS AND RISK FACTORS FOR OSTEOARTHRITIS

In the developed world, osteoarthritis of the knee is the biggest cause of chronic disability in the elderly. After the age of 55, more men suffer from hip osteoarthritis than women, while more women than men have osteoarthritis affecting the hands and knees. Before the age of 55, the distribution of osteoarthritis in the body is similar between the sexes. So far, nobody has been able to explain these distribution patterns between the sexes.

Race
Racial differences also exist. In Hong Kong, for example, the incidence of hip osteoarthritis is higher in the Caucasian population than in the Chinese population and in South Africa indigenous South Africans have a much lower incidence of hand and hip osteoarthritis than Caucasian South Africans. Whether the higher incidences in Caucasians in comparison with Asians and indigenous South Africans is genetically based or relates to joint usage is unknown.

Genetics
We do know that osteoarthritis follows in families. If you have a first degree relative (mother, father, brother or sister) with osteoarthritis, your risk of developing the condition is two to three times greater than if these relatives are unaffected. This is because DNA mutations lead to cartilage collagen protein abnormalities, which in turn can lead to the development of osteoarthritis.

Age
The most influential factor in the development of osteoarthritis is age. X-ray studies have shown 2 per cent of women under the age of 45 years, 30 per cent of women between 45 years and 65 years of age and 68 per cent of women older than 65 years have osteoarthritis. Figures for males are similar, although lower in the over 65s.

THE OLDER YOU GET, THE GREATER THE RISK OF DEVELOPING OSTEOARTHRITIS.

Joint trauma
The second most influential factor for the development of osteoarthritis is probably joint trauma, especially if the cartilage surface is damaged. The trauma can be a single major event, such as a fracture involving the joint (with accompanying joint surface disruption), or a cartilage tear. Trauma can also be the result of repetitive use of the joint particularly where the joint is overloaded. Although cartilage is resistant to damage in situations

of repeated movement, repetitive impact loads will lead to joint failure. Generally the earliest changes of osteoarthritis occur in a joint at the points that experience the greatest loads. This is why ballet dancers often get osteoarthritis of the ankle, baseball pitchers get it in the elbow and boxers get it in the knuckles when usually these are not common sites for osteoarthritis. In general, sport or physical exertion doesn't induce arthritis. The type of force that these people put on their joints is highly abnormal and it's the abnormality of the forces that's the problem. Long distance running and jogging have not been shown to induce osteoarthritis and there's no reason to stop sport because of the fear of developing arthritis.

Manual jobs where you have to repeatedly bend and lift can increase the risk of osteoarthritis of the lower spine, hips and knees because the abnormal dynamics of lifting repetitively will affect the weight-bearing joints. This doesn't mean a person without osteoarthritis shouldn't lift or bend, but you need to be aware that repetition can cause problems.

Obesity

Being overweight is another high risk factor for osteoarthritis, especially for severe osteoarthritis affecting the weight-bearing joints of the lower back, hips and knees. Even a small weight loss of only 5 kg means you can almost halve the risk of developing symptomatic osteoarthritis in the knee. If you're obese and don't already have osteoarthritis, you can reduce your risk by losing weight.

Sometimes an X-ray will show that your joints are badly affected by osteoarthritis, but surprisingly you don't show any symptoms. The reason you get pain in osteoarthritis is not well understood. For the knee joint, it appears that the amount of disability associated with osteoarthritis is related to how much wasting there is of the quadriceps muscle (the large muscle in the front of your thigh). It's not the amount of damage showing up on X-ray, or the amount of pain you're feeling. Also for a given set of osteoarthritic changes on X-ray, a woman will suffer more pain than a man in that joint.

CAUSES OF OSTEOARTHRITIS

Osteoarthritis usually has a primary cause—this means there are no predisposing factors (except genetics). Although the majority of secondary causes are related to joint trauma, there are many other secondary causes, including:

▶ congenital abnormalities such as unequal leg lengths or congenitally dislocated hips
▶ congenital metabolic diseases such as Wilson's disease (copper overload) or haemachromatosis (iron overload)
▶ endocrine diseases such as hyperthyroidism, diabetes, acromegaly (gigantism), hyperparathyroidism
▶ neuropathic abnormalities, where the nerve supply to the joint is damaged and you're unable to detect abnormal forces acting on the joint
▶ other forms of arthritis such as rheumatoid arthritis, which can damage a joint and lead to secondary osteoarthritis.

THE NATURE OF THE DISEASE

Osteoarthritis occurs in either of two ways. It can develop in joints with normal cartilage and bone, where the loads and stresses on the cartilage are excessive; or it can occur in joints where the loads would be considered reasonable but the cartilage and bone is abnormal, either because of previous damage to that area or because of congenital abnormalities.

Cartilage damage

Cartilage is a joint's main shock absorber, minimising a great deal of the concentrated force applied to it, preventing the bone from shattering. The other function of cartilage is to decrease the friction of movement within the joint. Most people who have anything to do with osteoarthritis believe the first changes of the disease occur in the load-bearing part of the cartilage.

Cartilage is produced by chondrocytes, the cells that make and lay down the two main substances of cartilage—proteoglycans, which gives the compressive stiffness to the tissue, allowing it to withstand loads, and collagen which provides tensile strength to withstand tearing. Cartilage also contains enzymes that break down bits of damaged cartilage.

In the early stages of osteoarthritis, the cartilage actually thickens because the arrangement and size of the collagen fibres becomes altered. As the abnormal forces acting on the joint continue, the glue network between the collagen fibres becomes permanently damaged. This damaged collagen is then fair game for the cartilage enzymes that have the job of removing

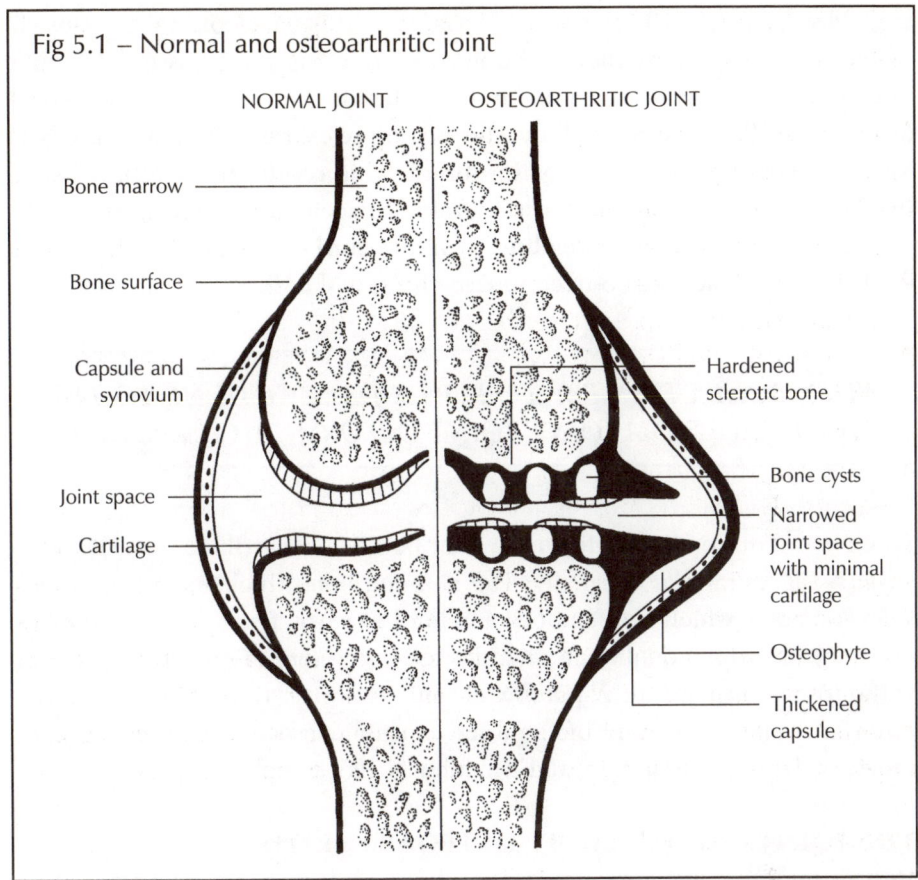

Fig 5.1 – Normal and osteoarthritic joint

NORMAL JOINT   OSTEOARTHRITIC JOINT

Bone marrow

Bone surface

Capsule and
synovium

Joint space

Cartilage

Hardened
sclerotic bone

Bone cysts

Narrowed
joint space
with minimal
cartilage

Osteophyte

Thickened
capsule

damaged cartilage, and the surface is softened and broken down. The
enzymes become overactive and damage continues to occur. Clefts
perpendicular to the cartilage surface then form and can turn into a deep
ulcer to the level of the bone. The damaged joint tries to repair itself but
the new cartilage is inferior to the original and can't stand up to
mechanical stresses to any great degree. With time, the continuing
damage to the cartilage results in the death of the chondrocytes, and
eventually all the cartilage in the mechanically used areas of the joint
disappears, resulting in bone rubbing on bone within the joint.

Bone damage

As well as cartilage damage within the joint, there's bone damage in
osteoarthritis. The bone cells try to repair damage done to the bone and
end up deforming the joint by producing bony spurring (osteophytes) on
the borders of the joint. These osteophytes interfere with functioning and
mobility and can even impinge on surrounding structures such as nerves

and blood vessels. The spine of the neck is susceptible to this if osteoarthritis develops there. The nerves supplying the arms can become pinched, causing pain and pins and needles in the arm, or the vertebral arteries can be compressed by the osteophytes resulting in decreased blood flow to the back part of the brain. This results in vertebro-basilar insufficiency, or mini-strokes to the brain. In accidents involving the neck, osteophytes can break off, leading to spinal cord compression and urgent surgery may be needed to decompress the spinal cord.

WHEN BONE CELLS TRY TO REPAIR DAMAGE DONE TO THE BONE AROUND A JOINT, JOINT DEFORMITY CAN RESULT.

When bone rubs on bone within the joint because of cartilage loss, the bone surface regenerates abnormally. The abraded bone thickens and becomes sclerotic bone, which is as smooth and hard as ivory. The sclerotic bone has no shock-absorbing quality at all and is the equivalent of operating your car without any suspension. A patchy, chronic synovitis (inflammation of the synovium) and thickening of the joint capsule can occur, decreasing joint mobility. Muscle wasting around the joint is also common.

THE JOINTS AFFECTED BY OSTEOARTHRITIS

Pain is the most obvious symptom of osteoarthritis—a deep ache localised in the joint. The pain is aggravated by joint use and relieved by rest and tends to be worse towards the end of the day, usually because you're more active during the day. If your osteoarthritis is particularly severe, the pain isn't relieved by rest and can continue through the night. Stiffness of the joint does occur but has its own features: it often occurs after rest but usually does not last longer than 15 minutes.

You may also experience 'gelling', a stiffness of the joint that only lasts a few seconds until you flex and extend the joint several times. It follows prolonged inactivity and is common in the elderly. A classic example is stiffness of the leg joints after getting out of a chair. The limitation of motion that occurs in osteoarthritis is because joint surfaces are not lined up appropriately, or because of muscle spasm, muscle wasting, joint capsule stiffening and shortening, or mechanical block from osteophytes or bits of cartilage that have broken off.

PAIN IS AGGRAVATED BY JOINT USE AND IS RELIEVED BY REST.

Although cartilage is the main site of destruction within an osteoarthritic joint, the cartilage itself isn't in pain, as it doesn't have any nerve pain fibres supplying it. This could explain why an X-ray may diagnose you as having severe osteoarthritis without you actually having any symptoms. The possible sites of pain in osteoarthritis include:

▶ the bone, where nerve fibres run along the outside covering of the bone and especially where new bone is laid down in osteophytes, stretching the nerve fibres
▶ microfractures of the bone below the cartilage
▶ congestion of blood vessels that are distorted by the physical changes within the osteoarthritic joint, or
▶ localised synovitis which can become as inflamed as the synovium in rheumatoid arthritis. (However, synovitis may actually be missing in a lot of cases of osteoarthritis.)

When you have your osteoarthritic joint examined it may show localised tenderness with associated soft tissue swelling. You'll probably get creaking and cracking when you move the joint since the bones, missing their cartilage, rub over one another. The muscles around the joint will also be wasted. In the advanced stages of osteoarthritis there is severe joint deformity with bony overgrowths (osteophytes) along the joint margins and quite possibly partial joint dislocation and limited range of joint movement.

Finger joints

Primary osteoarthritis usually affects the finger joints furthest away from the knuckles. It shows as Heberden's nodes or bony enlargements. They generally develop slowly with little or no pain, but can also progress rapidly often starting by minor trauma and resulting in acute severe pain and swelling. Your joint will usually have normal movement and function despite the deformity. Bouchard's nodes, however, are bony enlargements affecting the finger joints closest to the knuckles. The second most common site of primary osteoarthritis is the base of the thumb. The development of an osteophyte at this point of the hand results in a squared off appearance to the base of the thumb, often with pain, swelling and cracking at the joint when you move.

THE MOST COMMON SITES FOR PRIMARY ARTHRITIS ARE
THE FINGER JOINTS FURTHEST FROM THE KNUCKLE.

Hips

Most problems of the hip are secondary to congenital developmental problems of the hip. You might have only had minor problems early in life but later developed osteoarthritis. Up to 20 per cent of hip osteoarthritis is in both hips. You will usually only feel the pain in the groin, although you can also feel it in the buttocks, thigh or knee. Not being able to rotate the hip is an early sign of hip osteoarthritis. Try bringing your knee across your opposite thigh—if you find this difficult, it could be a warning sign.

Knees

The knee has three compartments and osteoarthritis can affect any or all of these. Usually, you will have bony deformity of the knee and if only the inside compartment of the knee is affected, the leg will become noticeably bowed. Your joint swells minimally with fluid and often creaks and cracks when you move. With knee osteoarthritis your quadriceps thigh muscle could also become wasted.

Spine

Osteoarthritis of the spine can involve either the discs between vertebrae or the facet joints at the side of the vertebrae (which help rotate the spine). If your doctor tells you you have spondylosis, your discs and joints between the vertebrae are affected by osteoarthritis. You will usually feel localised pain in the spine and will move stiffly. With progressive osteophyte formation two things can occur: nerve compression as the nerves come out of the bony canal of the spine or, more rarely, spinal cord compression.

INVESTIGATIONS INTO OSTEOARTHRITIS

Diagnosis of osteoarthritis is relatively simple if there are diagnostic X-ray changes. Your doctor needs to make sure the cause of the pain is actually the osteoarthritic joint (and not from somewhere else), as an osteoarthritic joint doesn't necessarily give you pain. Every doctor at some stage will get caught out with this—the classic case is a person with an osteoarthritic knee and hip complaining only of knee pain. It's not unnatural to assume that the knee is the problem, but 25 per cent of osteoarthritic hips present to the doctor with knee pain.

If there are no X-ray changes it is difficult to diagnose osteoarthritis. In these cases a technetium bone scan may show a diagnosis although you may have to resort to an invasive procedure, such as an arthroscopy, in which a telescope is inserted into the joint and the surgeon searches the joint looking for cartilage damage.

IF YOU HAVE KNEE PAIN YOU MAY HAVE
OSTEOARTHRITIS OF THE HIP.

Blood tests and aspiration of fluid from the joint are a waste of time with osteoarthritis, except in the initial stages of diagnosis to exclude other forms of arthritis. Diagnosis is based on what your doctor can see as well as X-ray findings. Typical X-ray findings of osteoarthritis are:

▶ a narrowing of the joint space between the bones of the joint, which in part is related to the loss of cartilage
▶ sclerosis of the bone (ivory-like, hardened, thickened) next to the joint
▶ cysts of the bone of the joint where the bone is destroyed and lost
▶ osteophyte development showing as bony spurs along the joint edge.

In later stages your doctor might also see partial dislocation of the joint.

TREATMENTS FOR OSTEOARTHRITIS
Treatment aims to decrease pain, maintain mobility and minimise disability. It's extremely important to decrease the load on an affected joint. If you know you're doing something that aggravates your osteoarthritis, stop, as it will only get worse. This is especially important if you're overweight and weight-bearing joints are involved. However complete rest of a joint is not a solution, as the joint will stiffen up and form a contracture.

Physical therapies
Physical therapies such as applying heat, massage, physiotherapy or hydrotherapy do provide relief. Strengthening the joint muscles will ease pain within several weeks, often at a level equivalent to non-steroidal anti-inflammatory medications.

Drug therapies
In comparison to inflammatory arthritis, there is only limited drug therapy

for the treatment of osteoarthritis. There are no potent disease-modifying drugs available, although glucosamine may improve cartilage structure. Analgesics work for pain relief, particularly simple analgesics, which are not addictive.

Don't take oral cortisone for osteoarthritis as the risk of side effects far outweighs any potential benefits. The action of non-steroidals in osteoarthritis is not well understood, although they do provide pain relief, especially during flare-ups, and make the joint more bearable. The general consensus is to use them in short bursts of seven to 10 days at a time when the joint is playing up and to stop use once it has settled down. Continuous use is usually not recommended as it increases the risk of side effects, but is sometimes unavoidable. Injecting the joint with cortisone or Synvisc are stop-gap measures to try to delay surgery.

Surgery

Osteotomies, arthroscopies and joint replacements are surgeries you could consider as surgery does have a lot to offer for pain relief and improved joint function in moderate to severe forms of osteoarthritis (See Chapter 2).

DISH

DISH, or Diffuse Idiopathic Skeletal Hyperostosis is thought to be a variant of osteoarthritis, although it appears not to affect cartilaginous joints. There is severe calcification and bony changes in the ligaments that run down the sides of the spine. On X-ray it looks like wax has run down the side of the spine, just as hot wax runs down the side of a candle. Although DISH can involve the whole spine, it's often restricted to the middle and bottom of the spine and is usually seen in older people.

Despite the extensive abnormalities seen on X-ray, you will often only have mild pain and your mobility only moderately affected. DISH can also cause irregular new bone formation at the back of the elbow, the base of the heel and at the kneecap. The main symptoms of DISH are restricted spinal movements with prominent spinal stiffness. You can have pain in the spine as well as at other affected sites. If the neck spine is affected, nerve compression is common and heel pain from the development of a bony spur is also common.

DISH is associated with diabetes and high blood sugar levels with twice the levels that are seen in population studies of people without DISH. Why this is so is not known and neither is the cause of DISH. People with DISH also have high vitamin A levels, so if you're being treated with high dose retinoids, a synthetic vitamin A-like compound for certain skin diseases, you can develop DISH-like abnormalities. Whether or not high levels of vitamin A in the body stimulate the development of DISH needs further research. The treatment for DISH is the same as for osteoarthritis.

WHAT TO EXPECT

As you grow older, you'll not necessarily develop a disability from osteoarthritis. The disease often stabilises, especially if you make sure you don't excessively load a joint. You may even find there's a reversal of the disease with decreasing pain and the X-ray changes of osteoarthritis may reverse. The outlook is variable. Because osteoarthritis doesn't have any other effects on the body and is restricted in its effects to the joint involved, there is no change to your life expectancy with this disease.

CHAPTER | 6

RHEUMATOID ARTHRITIS

Rheumatoid arthritis is a disease that affects not only joints, but many organs of the body. You will usually also have an inflammatory synovitis—inflammation of the synovial layer around a joint—causing that joint to become tender and swollen. The synovitis particularly affects the small joints of your limbs. This inflammation leads to bone erosion and cartilage destruction, which damage and deform the joints.

The destructive element of the disease varies and may range from a brief episode affecting only one or two joints to widespread arthritis that becomes chronic. A blood test for an antibody, rheumatoid factor, can give some indication of the severity of disease activity—the higher the levels of rheumatoid factor, the more severe the disease. You're unlikely to have the aggressive disease unless you're older or have high levels of the rheumatoid factor. If you have rheumatoid arthritis with normal levels of rheumatoid factor, you'll usually fare better and have a less severe disease.

---

*THE HANDS ARE THE MOST COMMON SITE OF
RHEUMATOID ARTHRITIS—THE JOINTS BECOME
INFLAMED, SWOLLEN AND PAINFUL.*

STATISTICS AND RISK FACTORS FOR RHEUMATOID ARTHRITIS

There are approximately 250,000 people in Australia with rheumatoid arthritis—about eight people in every one thousand. Women are three times more likely to be afflicted than men. The risk of rheumatoid arthritis increases with age, but as we age, there are likely to be fewer differences in the disease between men and women. Eighty per cent of sufferers of rheumatoid arthritis will have an onset of their disease between the ages of 35 to 50 years of age.

Genetics

As with osteoarthritis, there is a family predisposition to rheumatoid arthritis and if you have a first degree relative (mother, father, brother or sister) with the disease, the risk of you developing rheumatoid arthritis is increased four times. This has been confirmed in studies of identical twins, although genetic studies are still confusing as there are at least six different genes associated with rheumatoid arthritis, and different genes predominate in different ethnic groups.

It's also possible that different genes as well as multiple susceptible genes influence how severe and destructive the rheumatoid arthritis will be. Genetic studies show a genetic predisposition to toxic reactions with certain drugs used to treat rheumatoid arthritis. Genetic predispositions still need to have an environmental trigger to set off the disease. So as well as finding the genetic map of rheumatoid arthritis and the genetic map for drug reactions in rheumatoid arthritis, we also still need to find the trigger, which could be ingested toxins, infections, climate, urban versus rural living, the hole in the ozone layer or something else.

CAUSES OF RHEUMATOID ARTHRITIS

The cause of rheumatoid arthritis is still unknown. Because the disease occurs worldwide, the cause would be common everywhere, and is probably something infectious that triggers the disease in those people genetically susceptible to it. At different times *mycoplasma*, Epstein-Barr virus (glandular fever), cytomegalovirus, rubella virus (German measles) and *parvovirus* have been thought to cause rheumatoid arthritis. It has also been speculated that one of these infections—or another germ—releases a *super-antigen*, or toxin, which adheres to a gene permanently. This would lead to stimulation of the immune system resulting in rheumatoid arthritis. However a lot more work needs to be done before a final genetic theory and triggering factor are proven to be the cause of rheumatoid arthritis.

DOCTORS AND SCIENTISTS BELIEVE THAT SOMETHING INFECTIOUS TRIGGERS RHEUMATOID ARTHRITIS IN PEOPLE WHO ARE GENETICALLY SUSCEPTIBLE TO IT.

THE NATURE OF THE DISEASE
The earliest damage in rheumatoid arthritis is injury to the small blood vessels supplying the synovium, and an associated increase in the number of synovial cells. As the process progresses, the number of inflammatory cells around the small blood vessels increases, resulting in further inflammation with fluid, swelling and pain in the joint. The major inflammatory cells are:

▶ macrophages which are large scavenger cells that clean up cell debris and chemically attack perceived germs (normal cells) around the joint aggressively.
▶ white blood cells called T lymphocytes which release chemicals that attack the surrounding tissue
▶ white blood cells called B lymphocytes which release antibodies involved in signposting germs (or body cells mistaken for germs)
▶ synovial fibroblasts which release chemicals that can degrade joint tissues and cartilage.

These four groups of cells infiltrate the joint tissues, especially the synovium and synovial fluid, leading to the inflammation and swelling of rheumatoid arthritis. The synovium then grows over into the joint cavity. The synovial covering of the joint surface leads to joint damage, especially to the cartilage and bone, resulting in a typical rheumatoid joint in which a lot of the swelling has a 'boggy', rather than fluid, feel to it. Doctors refer to this boggy synovial swelling as a *pannus* to differentiate it from other types of swelling associated with different types of arthritis.

The rheumatoid pannus contains chemicals that have been secreted by the inflammatory cells. These chemicals account for many of the manifestations of rheumatoid arthritis, including inflammation of the synovium and synovial fluid, synovial overgrowth, cartilage and bone damage, in addition to rheumatoid problems away from the joints, including malaise and fatigue. Inflammatory chemicals released into the blood stream from the synovium result in rheumatoid manifestations in your organs. These chemicals are interleukins, interferons, granulocyte colony stimulating factors, tumour necrosis factor, macrophage colony stimulating factor, platelet growth factor, and insulin-like growth factor. They also lead to the release of other inflammatory chemicals such as histamine, collagenase and prostaglandins. As you can see, the chemistry of rheumatoid arthritis is dauntingly complex.

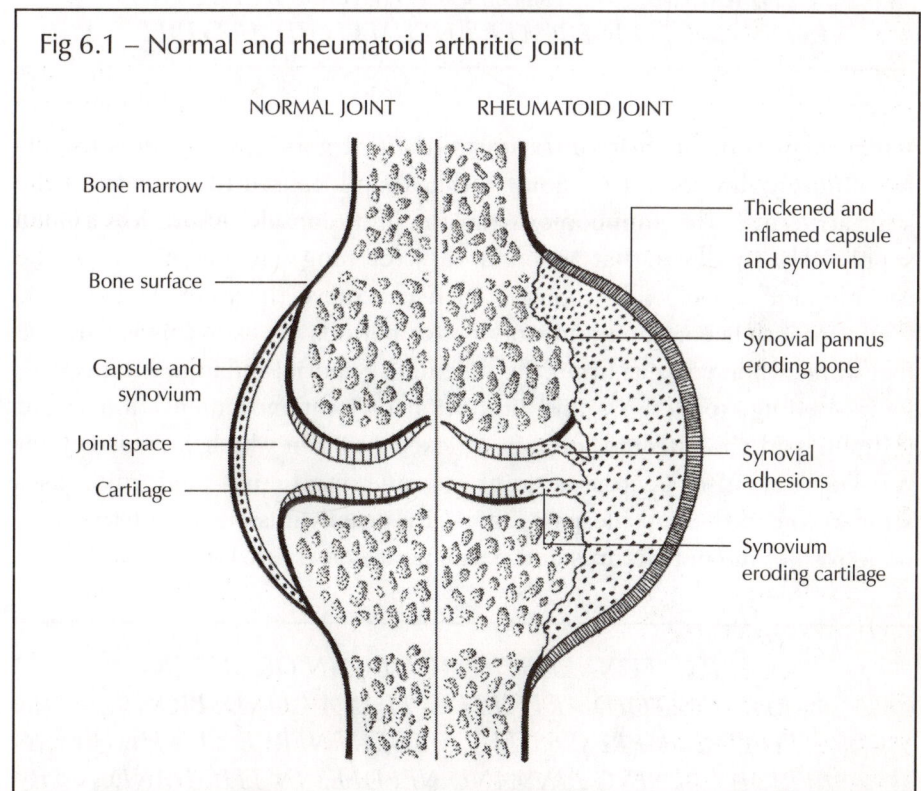

Fig 6.1 – Normal and rheumatoid arthritic joint

NORMAL JOINT   RHEUMATOID JOINT

Bone marrow

Bone surface

Capsule and synovium

Joint space

Cartilage

Thickened and inflamed capsule and synovium

Synovial pannus eroding bone

Synovial adhesions

Synovium eroding cartilage

FEATURES OF RHEUMATOID ARTHRITIS

Rheumatoid arthritis usually starts insidiously. Two thirds of people start off by experiencing fatigue, loss of appetite, weight loss, generalised weakness and vague aches and pains. It feels like the flu and your doctor might think that's what it is until the inflammation of the joint becomes obvious. These symptoms can last several months and its difficult to diagnose rheumatoid arthritis before the joints flare up.

Hands, fingers, wrists, knees, feet and toes are especially affected in rheumatoid arthritis, as well as both sides of the body. This symmetry of distribution is typical of rheumatoid arthritis. It is also typical to find it affects four or more joints. In about 10 per cent of people the onset is very rapid and aggressive—arthritis of the joints is widespread, fevers are usually around 38°C, and the lymph nodes and spleen are enlarged.

FATIGUE, LOSS OF APPETITE, WEIGHT LOSS, GENERALISED WEAKNESS AND VAGUE ACHES AND PAINS COULD INDICATE RHEUMATOID ARTHRITIS.

When rheumatoid arthritis first starts to affect a joint, the pain is usually felt diffusely throughout the joint rather than localised to one part of the joint structure. The pain comes from the joint capsule, which has a good supply of pain fibres that respond to stretching and distension of the capsule, and is especially aggravated if you move the joint. Generalised joint stiffness is common and worse after periods of rest—this is why you feel worse when you get up in the morning. Synovial inflammation causes joint swelling, tenderness and limitation of joint movement. You might initially hold the affected joint in a flexed position which increases joint volume, but also decreases joint capsule stretching and minimises stimulation of the capsule pain fibres. Eventually, fusion of soft tissue or bone results in contractures and permanent deformities of the joint.

CARPAL TUNNEL SYNDROME CAN OCCUR IN RHEUMATOID ARTHRITIS. IT IS A CONDITION THAT COMPRESSES THE MEDIAN NERVE AT THE WRIST, CAUSING PINS AND NEEDLES IN THE HAND.

Your hands are the most likely area to be affected, especially the finger joints closest to the knuckle, the wrist and the knuckle itself. For some unknown reason, the finger joints furthest from the knuckles seem to be spared. Synovial swelling at the wrist can often lead to compression of the median nerve at the wrist which gives you pins and needles in the index and middle fingers as well as some loss of function of the hand in the parts supplied by the median nerve. Known as carpal tunnel syndrome, you may need surgery to correct this.

Rheumatoid arthritis often affects knees and you'll usually have synovial swelling, chronic fluid on the knee and knee ligament laxity. You may only feel pain at the back of the knee where an overgrowth of synovium and synovial fluid accumulation results in a swelling known as a Baker's cyst. Rheumatoid arthritis affecting the ankle, forefeet and balls of the feet can lead to rapid immobilisation and foot deformities.

The most common part of the spine to be involved is the neck, but rarely, if ever, the lower spine. Rheumatoid arthritis of the neck can give you intractable headaches and even migraines. Rarely, the destruction of the joints in the necks by rheumatoid arthritis can lead to an unstable spine and compression of the spinal cord. This needs urgent surgery to re-stabilise the neck.

Joint deformities
Rheumatoid arthritis can lead to joint deformities, especially of the hands and wrists, including:

▶ partial dislocation of the wrists in which the wrist bones drop away from the ulna bone of the forearm, leaving an *ulna subluxation* or step;
▶ *ulna deviation* of the fingers at the knuckle joints so that when you look at the palm of your hand, the fingers point inwards;
▶ *swan-neck* deformity of the fingers in which over-straightening of the finger joints closest to the knuckles and compensatory over-bending of the finger joints furthest from the knuckles occurs; and
▶ *z-plasty* deformity of the thumbs in which there is over-bending of the joint between the thumb and hand and over-straightening of the thumb joint itself, forming a 'z' shape to the thumb and resulting in a loss of thumb mobility and pinch grip.

You can also get similar destructive deformities in the feet (both the hands and feet are especially affected by deformities). These are precipitated by laxity of the supporting soft tissues of the joints, destruction and weakening of ligaments, tendons and the joint capsule, muscle imbalance and unopposed forces acting on the joints of the hands when you use your hands. If they are affected by inflammation, the tendons become weakened and if you use too much force, the tendon can rupture and you might need tendon repair or even tendon grafting.

Rheumatoid arthritis affects the whole body and those manifestations that don't involve a joint are known as extra-articular manifestations. These tend to occur if you have severe, aggressive arthritis and are infrequent in most people with rheumatoid.

Rheumatoid nodules

Rheumatoid nodules, which occur in about 30 per cent of sufferers, are swellings that occur away from joints and are often in areas of mechanical pressure, such as on the back of the forearms and hands, although they can also occur in non-mechanical areas such as in the lung and lining of the brain. They vary in size and consistency and are thought to originate in areas of blood vessel inflammation resulting first in the loss of blood to the surrounding tissue and then the tissue dying off. The body's response to dead tissue is to isolate it by surrounding it with inflammatory cells, which enclose the tissue from the rest of the body. You will rarely get symptoms from rheumatoid nodules but they can become infected or traumatised and are unsightly.

Muscle wasting

You may notice muscle weakness and wasting (which is common) soon after your arthritis starts. This usually happens in the muscles close to affected joints, especially the hands. The small hand muscles that lie between the bones often waste away, leaving 'gutters' between the bones.

Inflammation of blood vessels

Vasculitis, or inflammation of blood vessels, can appear within any organ in the body—the consequences depend on which organ is affected. Vasculitis usually affects the smaller arteries. When the blood vessel becomes inflamed, the blood supply to the organ supplied by that vessel is cut off as the blood vessel becomes swollen and breaks down. That part of the organ then dies. If the artery supplies the finger or toes the digit can become gangrenous. If the artery is supplying the brain or heart, you could have a stroke or heart attack. If the kidneys are affected you can develop renal failure. Fortunately, however, involvement of the heart, brain and kidneys is rare. Nerve paralysis can occur if the blood supply to a nerve is affected.

No organ in the body is immune to this process but widespread vasculitis is rare. Limited forms are, however, common and the vasculitis is directly related to higher levels of rheumatoid factor in the blood, an indicator of disease activity. For some reason, people of African descent are not likely to develop rheumatoid vasculitis.

Inflammation of the lung

Your lungs are more likely to be affected if you're a man, and symptoms could include:

▶ a pleurisy-like inflammation of the lining of the lung
▶ inflammation of the arteries of the lung giving a form of vasculitis
▶ the formation of rheumatoid nodules that rupture the lung tissue
▶ a pneumonia-like (non-infectious) inflammation of the lung tissue, which might cause extreme scarring leading to possible fibrosis and making you look like a smoker with emphysema.

Rheumatoid damage to the lung can also make you more prone to lung infections because of damage to the lung's structure and local immune system.

With rheumatoid arthritis, although lung problems are common, you'll rarely have symptoms.

Rheumatoid arthritis and the heart

Your heart can be affected by rheumatoid arthritis, but fortunately symptoms from it are rare. The pericardium (the fibrous sack surrounding the heart) is the site most commonly affected, occurring in 50 per cent of people with rheumatoid. Rarely the pericardium will become scarred or fill with fluid and limit the output from the heart resulting in heart failure.

Eye damage

Sjogren's syndrome (see Chapter 11) occurs in up to 20 per cent of people and happens when there is damage to the lacrimal gland of the eye, which produces tears. Tears carry important nutrients to the cornea, or window to the eye, as the cornea doesn't have a blood supply. (If the cornea had a blood supply it would be opaque as blood vessels would obscure our vision.) Without tears the cornea becomes inflamed and cloudy resulting in a red, irritated eye with eventual loss of vision. Luckily the cure is simply putting nutrient drops in your eye four or five times a day, to replace what the body no longer produces. Less than 1 per cent of people have problems that affect the eye's deeper structures. Scleritis, an inflammation of the white of the eye, is due to a rheumatoid nodule-like lesion affecting the sclera— if left untreated it can lead to rupture of the eyeball.

Other problems
Felty's syndrome is an uncommon manifestation that is more likely to happen if you have a long-standing disease. The spleen enlarges, and you will have suppressed bone marrow with low white blood cell counts and occasionally anaemia and bleeding problems. These patients often have quite severe rheumatoid arthritis with high levels of rheumatoid factor in the blood and a lot of extra-articular manifestations of the disease. Because of the abnormalities of the spleen and bone marrow, if you have Felty's syndrome, you're prone to catching infections and can quickly become sick. If you have rheumatoid arthritis you should be immunised for as many diseases as is reasonable, including influenza and pneumonia.

Osteoporosis, secondary to rheumatoid arthritis, is common even if you're not taking cortisone for treatment, and seems to be related to the degree of inflammation. There's a moderate risk of bone fractures from osteoporosis and the bone mass can be improved with exercise and bone preserving medications such as calcitriol, palmidronate, alendronate and etidronate.

INVESTIGATIONS INTO RHEUMATOID ARTHRITIS
The final diagnosis of rheumatoid arthritis is based on what the doctor sees. A blood test can confirm the diagnosis, but the problem with measuring levels of rheumatoid factor is that it's not specific to rheumatoid arthritis and can be raised in other types of inflammatory diseases, such as systemic lupus erythematosus (see Chapter 8), chronic liver disease, and even syphilis and tuberculosis. Another complication is that rheumatoid factor occurs in 5 per cent of the normal, healthy population without any history or symptoms of rheumatoid arthritis and increases in the normal population with ageing—up to 20 per cent of people over 65 years of age are positive for rheumatoid factor without having the disease. And it is only positive in about two-thirds of cases.

If it looks like you have classic rheumatoid arthritis but have a negative blood test for rheumatoid factor you're said to have sero-negative rheumatoid arthritis.

So rheumatoid factor doesn't necessarily mean you have rheumatoid arthritis, but if you have negative levels on blood tests, or sero-negative arthritis, you generally have a much more favourable outcome than someone with a positive rheumatoid factor in their blood.

Other routine blood tests in the initial stages of diagnosis include a full blood count (FBC) to check for anaemia, low white blood cells and platelet numbers (low platelet counts may indicate potential bleeding problems). Your doctor will do an erthrocyte sedimentation rate (ESR) both initially and as part of follow-up monitoring. This is a cheap and reasonably accurate indicator of disease activity, which increases in nearly all people with active rheumatoid arthritis. Instead of an ESR, your doctor might do a c-reactive protein or ceruloplasmin level to show disease activity (although these are less popular, due to their cost).

BLOOD TESTS FOR RHEUMATOID ARTHRITIS
INCLUDE RHEUMATOID FACTOR AND ESR.

If your joint is swollen with fluid it's possible to simply aspirate fluid from the joint with a needle and then test it for rheumatoid factor and white blood cell levels. If your doctor isn't certain of the diagnosis, the fluid can be examined for other features, such as the presence of crystals for gout (see Chapter 13), to exclude other potential diagnoses.

In the initial stages of diagnosing rheumatoid arthritis, X-rays don't help as they show normal joints and bones and swollen soft tissue around the joint—both obvious to the naked eye. As the disease progresses, X-rays will show changes that indicate rheumatoid arthritis. However, if you've been treated effectively, these changes of disease progression will appear on subsequent X-rays. This indicates that the disease is being well controlled by your medication, as the levels of changes showing up on X-ray will, like the appearance of rheumatoid factor, give a reasonable idea of how your disease is progressing. The changes are osteopaenia (loss of calcium) in the bone near the joints, and erosions of the bone of the joint caused by the pannus overlying the joint surface releasing chemicals that destroy the bone. Other methods of imaging the joints, such as technetium bone scans and magnetic resonance imaging (MRI), are expensive and aren't usually warranted, as they'll be unlikely to lead to a change in diagnosis.

If your symptoms are slow to start and don't involve your joints, it may take time to reach a diagnosis. According to some texts, the average delay in diagnosis after disease onset is about nine months. This is because not all cases are clear-cut—some cases may take up to two years to become obvious. Some of the early symptoms may also not be bad enough to make you seek medical help. As the disease progresses, diagnosis becomes easier. The American College of Rheumatology has published revised criteria to help diagnose rheumatoid arthritis. Four of the following seven criteria need to be met for you to be classified as having rheumatoid arthritis.

1. Joint stiffness is present in the mornings and lasts longer than one hour.
2. Arthritis affects three or more defined joint areas.
3. Arthritis affects either the wrists, the knuckle, or the finger joints closest to the knuckle.
4. The arthritis is symmetrical, affecting the same joints on both sides of the body.
5. Rheumatoid nodules are present.
6. There is an elevated rheumatoid factor in the blood or synovial fluid.
7. X-ray changes are consistent with rheumatoid arthritis (as previously described).

IT CAN TAKE UP TO NINE MONTHS FROM
THE ONSET OF THE DISEASE TO BE DIAGNOSED
WITH RHEUMATOID ARTHRITIS.

TREATMENT OF RHEUMATOID ARTHRITIS

Treatment aims to minimise symptoms and slow down the destruction of joints and other organs of the body. None of the current treatment regimes will cure your arthritis, but many are good at switching the disease off and preventing further damage. You need a multi-disciplinary approach involving physiotherapists, occupational therapists, podiatrists and psychologists if necessary. You may not need to see all these therapists, but their input sooner rather than later can improve your outcome.

Drug therapy

Simple analgesics or narcotic analgesics will give you pain relief. Non-steroidal anti-inflammatory medications or low dose cortisone medications, can also improve pain, stiffness and joint mobility. Disease-modifying drugs include methotrexate, sulfasalazine, penicillamine, gold, hydroxychloroquine, azathioprine, cyclosporin and possibly cortisone. You can use these drugs by themselves or in combination depending on how bad your rheumatoid arthritis is and how it responds to medications.

Once you stop using the drugs, remissions are infrequent, although some of the literature suggests remissions don't happen at all and that the disease will recur rapidly after you stop taking medication. The current most popular disease-modifying drug is methotrexate because it's more rapid in its onset of action, less toxic and you can use it for longer periods of time.

Surgery

The role of surgery in rheumatoid arthritis is usually confined to trying to improve the function of severely damaged joints. Joint replacements for the hips and knees are more successful than shoulder joint replacements. It is important to have realistic goals—surgery is not intended to give you a normal joint, but to improve joint pain and function. Reconstructive hand surgery will give a better cosmetic effect, which may be important for your self-image, and your hand function may also be improved. Reconstructive hand surgery is highly specialised so if you need it, find the most qualified surgeon you can.

WHAT TO EXPECT

The vast majority of people with rheumatoid arthritis will not suffer major problems but if several of the following points apply to you, then you're more likely to have an aggessive disease with joint destruction:

▶ the presence of more than 20 inflamed joints
▶ a very high ESR
▶ high levels of rheumatoid factor in the blood
▶ X-ray evidence of joint erosions
▶ the presence of rheumatoid nodules
▶ persistent inflammation
▶ advanced age at onset
▶ presence of other medical conditions
▶ lower socio-economic group
▶ the presence of the HLA-DRB10401 and HLA-DRB0404 genes.

If several of these apply to you, you're more likely to have an aggressive disease.

Rheumatoid arthritis tends to have a variable outcome. If you've had sustained disease activity for more than a year, it doesn't necessarily mean it will get worse at the same rate of progression. The greatest amount of joint damage actually occurs in the first 12 months of the disease, compared with the second and third years. Fifty per cent of people will develop joint erosions within the first year of their disease and foot joints are affected more frequently than hand joints. If you start treatment quickly this can be stopped. Functional disability develops maximally in the first two years and thereafter follows any X-ray change. If no bone erosions show on X-ray, joint function needs to be maintained. The more bone erosions on X-ray, the greater the functional disability. Generally you will find the arthritis is worse in the first six years, after which it slows down.

Your average life expectancy with rheumatoid arthritis is shortened by three to seven years, but seems to be limited to those with severe joint disease and associated vasculitis. Disease-modifying drug therapy can help, as it is intended to decrease the disease activity, the risk of joint deformities and extra-articular manifestations occurring, as well as improve quality of life.

JUVENILE RHEUMATOID ARTHRITIS

D espite its name, juvenile rheumatoid arthritis can affect both adults and children. Although it isn't immunologically the same as adult-onset rheumatoid arthritis, there are some features that are similar to the adult disease. Also known as Still's Disease after George Frederick Still who first described it in 1897, the disease is not common and generally has a favourable outcome.

Juvenile rheumatoid arthritis can be hard to diagnose as its onset can be extremely variable. There are many symptoms and manifestations. Some reports suggest errors in initial diagnosis occur in up to half the cases that present to specialists because the initial presentation is unlikely to be 'classic'. Sometimes the diagnosis is only arrived at after the elimination of the many other possible causes of the symptoms. To further confuse the issue it can even present in a child just an unexplained fever and manifestations that are unrelated to the joints. It can also occur in adults—the oldest known person to suffer juvenile rheumatoid arthritis was 70 years of age at first presentation. So much for its name! Maybe it should be called 'not juvenile not rheumatoid not arthritis'.

THERE ARE MANY VARYING SYMPTOMS AND MANIFESTATIONS OF JUVENILE RHEUMATOID ARTHRITIS.

STATISTICS AND CAUSES OF JUVENILE RHEUMATOID ARTHRITIS

Juvenile rheumatoid arthritis is rare before the age of six months and usually starts between the ages of one and three years or eight and 12 years. Girls are twice as likely to get the disease as boys.

The cause is unknown, although there are many theories. Infections with the bacteria *streptococcus*, which usually occur in the throat, have been assumed to be involved because of raised markers in the blood, but these markers are non-specific and occur in other diseases as well. Rubella, or German measles, has also been named as the culprit but, again, there is little evidence to support this.

THE CAUSE OF JUVENILE RHEUMATOID ARTHRITIS IS UNKNOWN.

Other cited factors are upper respiratory infections, trauma and emotional stress. It's difficult to assess these factors—emotional upset aggravates any illness, and if you're suffering with a disease you may be emotional anyway, so it's more likely that emotional stresses are secondary to the arthritis rather than the cause.

Your genes play a part in the development of most inflammatory illnesses and a correlation has been found between the HLA-B27 genetic marker and juvenile rheumatoid arthritis. As with rheumatoid arthritis, there are also other elevated markers found in juvenile rheumatoid arthritis, but more clarification is needed before a conclusion can be made.

INVESTIGATIONS INTO JUVENILE RHEUMATOID ARTHRITIS

There are no specific blood markers for juvenile rheumatoid arthritis.

Unlike the adult variety, a positive rheumatoid factor is not common at all and is present in only 10 to 20 per cent of cases. However, a positive rheumatoid factor often indicates a poorer outlook for joint movement and use. A non-specific marker, the anti-nuclear antibody, is positive in up to 50 per cent of cases, but this marker is so non-specific it only indicates that something is wrong, without saying what. Your doctor will reach a diagnosis of juvenile rheumatoid arthritis by doing blood tests to exclude different forms of arthritis.

If your immunoglobulin levels are elevated, this is a marker for more aggressive disease. High levels of immunoglobulins are associated with poorer joint function and the hip is more likely to be attacked by the disease.

Your doctor may order other blood tests to get an idea of severity of the disease. The erthrocyte sedimentation rate (ESR) is a good indicator of disease activity as well as how you might respond to treatment. With the full blood count (FBC) you may have a low-grade anaemia, which improves with treatment, and a raised white cell count showing the increased risk of extra-articular features.

Analysis of synovial fluid gives variable results and often the severity of the disease is not indicated by them. But it's a good way of excluding arthritis caused by an infection, so if the joint is easily accessible and your doctor isn't certain of the analysis, this is helpful to do.

X-rays are not usually helpful except to exclude other possible causes of the symptoms. It's only later in the disease that X-rays will show features consistent with juvenile rheumatoid arthritis such as bone erosions and loss of calcium around the joint.

FEATURES OF JUVENILE RHEUMATOID ARTHRITIS

Juvenile rheumatoid arthritis is usually indicated by remissions and flare-ups of large and small joint arthritis with associated disturbances in growth. There may also be high fevers, enlarged lymph nodes, enlarged spleen, enlarged liver, pleurisy and inflammation of the pericardium (the sac around the heart).

There are three types of presentation for juvenile rheumatoid arthritis— systemic (whole body), pauciarticular (arthritis affecting up to four joints) and polyarticular (arthritis affecting five or more joints). Each onset type has its own hazards.

Systemic presentation

High, spiking fevers, a fairly typical rash, enlarged lymph nodes, enlarged spleen, and heart, brain and lung involvement are characteristic of this type. Despite the seriousness of the disease and how widespread it is, you may only have pain without any swelling and stiffness (which indicates severe arthritis) in your joints. The two major hazards are convulsions due to brain irritation or heart failure from inflammation of the heart muscle. About 20 per cent of people with juvenile rheumatoid arthritis have the systemic type, and more boys are more affected by this type than girls. If there is an active arthritis, the diagnosis is straightforward; if you have only minor joint aches the diagnosis can be trickier. A younger child usually appears listless, sick and irritable with possible loss of appetite and weight loss. Despite high fevers, older children may look well and they may have fevers for several months before any arthritis develops.

FEVERS, RASH, LOSS OF APPETITE AND WEIGHT LOSS CAN BE INDICATORS OF JUVENILE RHEUMATOID ARTHRITIS.

Joints aren't always affected in juvenile rheumatoid arthritis, but if your child has joint pain, he or she may prefer to be inactive, even avoiding walking. Children also tend to protect a joint from pain by keeping it bent—you can see this in their posture and sleeping position.

Up to 90 per cent of people with the systemic type have a rash. This can be in discrete patches or it may join together into wider areas over your whole body, including the soles of the feet and palms of the hands. In most children the rash is non-itchy, but it can get worse with a fever. You might also see variations in the degree of redness, especially if you apply heat or light pressure or rub the skin.

The heart complication of the systemic type can be serious—even fatal in a small percentage of children—and may give symptoms of shortness of breath, rapid breathing and a rapid heart rate. The sac surrounding the heart can get inflamed but this isn't usually serious. The lungs may be inflamed either independently or along with the heart. Enlargement of the spleen is common, enlargement of the liver less so, but if these organs do enlarge, you may get pain in your stomach or feel bloated. The liver, spleen, kidneys and heart can be hit by secondary amyloidosis, a condition in which these organs' cells are replaced with the protein amyloid, which is overproduced in some diseases with chronic inflammation. Although this condition can be fatal and accounts for the majority of deaths with juvenile rheumatoid arthritis, deaths are rare.

Pauciarticular presentation

Four or fewer joints ar affected with this type of juvenile rheumatoid arthritis. Affecting girls more often than boys, it accounts for 40 to 50 per cent of people with juvenile rheumatoid arthritis. The arthritis is slow and creeping to begin and may be mild. Fevers are usually low grade, but young children are often listless, irritable and don't grow at a normal rate. The heart and lungs are never affected and the biggest hazard is inflammation of the eye, iridocyclitis, which leads to loss of vision. It can occur months to years before the arthritis starts.

Polyarticular presentation

Severe joint deformity as the arthritis progresses is characteristic of this third type of juvenile rheumatoid arthritis. Five or more joints are affected and the disease may develop either slowly or rapidly. This type accounts for 30 per cent to 40 per cent of children with juvenile rheumatoid arthritis with girls most affected. Children usually look ill and also may have fevers, loss of appetite and weight loss. The large joints are affected initially and are usually swollen and tender with restricted range of movement. The small joints of the hands and feet may be affected, and the condition may be symmetrical across the body or may migrate between the sides of the body. The hips and neck are also frequently affected, as well as the joints between the jaw and skull.

In juvenile rheumatoid arthritis, as with rheumatoid arthritis, nodules sometimes form below the skin which means the disease is more aggressive and deforming. Nodules occur mostly on the back of the forearms, elbows and the back of the heels. Some children with the polyarticular form of juvenile rheumatoid arthritis, experience early fusion of the bone growth plates resulting in shortened stature, a stiff, straightened neck, small hands and feet and shortening of the jaw. This is only permanent if the disease activity is prolonged and unremitting. In general, once the disease becomes less aggressive and goes into remission your child's growth will continue normally.

TREATMENT OF JUVENILE RHEUMATOID ARTHRITIS

The treatments offered for juvenile rheumatoid arthritis depend on which type you or your child has. If there is substantial evidence of a systemic presentation, your doctor will usually take an aggressive approach to treatment, especially because of the small mortality risk due to the disease's potential to affect major organs. The primary aim is to relieve suffering. There is no reason to leave your child in pain—and simple analgesics may not be enough. Aspirin or other non-steroidal anti-inflammatory drugs are recommended for children in pain.

The next step is to find an acceptable disease-modifying agent such as methotrexate, gold and salazopyrin. Although these medications are potent, the risks of the disease can far outweigh the risks of a drug's side effects. Cortisone, as well as arthritis itself, can make you shorter in stature. Yet cortisone rapidly gives symptom relief and also blocks disease progression.

YOUNG PEOPLE WITH JUVENILE RHEUMATOID ARTHRITIS NEED TO ADAPT TO THE ONGOING NATURE OF THEIR DISEASE. PROFESSIONAL PSYCHOLOGISTS MAY BE ABLE TO HELP.

Once the disease activity has been switched off and your child gets relief from symptoms, he or she needs help to come to terms with this lifelong disease. This is especially so if the major organs have been affected or there is a possibility of deformation. Juvenile rheumatoid arthritis can place limitations on life and major psychological adjustments are needed. Professional psychological help may be of great value. Most hospitals have child and adolescent units that have child psychologists available to help if needed.

WHAT TO EXPECT

Studies have shown that complete remission occurs in 50 per cent of people who develop juvenile rheumatoid arthritis. A further 20 per cent in full remission regain full function, although they still have the disease. Remission can occur at any time. Infrequently, a child's disease which has gone into remission may flare up again in adulthood leading to joint destruction for the first time. Most children who develop juvenile rheumatoid arthritis will keep having attacks and remissions but only a small percentage of children get progressively worse. The survival rate of children with severe systemic juvenile rheumatoid arthritis is very high. The small percentage of children who do die (2 to 4 per cent) have prolonged polyarthritis with secondary infection, secondary amyloidosis or heart failure.

CHAPTER | 8

SYSTEMIC LUPUS ERYTHEMATOSUS

L upus erythematosus is Latin for 'whole body red wolf'. Systemic lupus erythematosus is a disease associated with a red rash and which aggressively destroys body organs. As with most forms of inflammatory arthritis, it affects the whole body and is not restricted to joints. Up to 90 per cent of cases occur in women and particularly those of child-bearing age, but it can occasionally affect the elderly and children. It significantly reduces life expectancy.

CAUSES OF SYSTEMIC LUPUS ERYTHEMATOSUS

The actual cause of lupus is still unknown. It's thought to have a different cause from rheumatoid arthritis because the obvious features of the two diseases are different, as well as the immune markers in the blood. The combination of immune markers, immune white blood cell actions and the inadequate regulation of these immune reactions by the body means tissue is destroyed. It's thought that the combination of genetic predisposition and unknown environmental factors, such as chemicals or infections, trigger these immune reactions.

Genetics

Lupus has a genetic link. Approximately 40 per cent of identical twins will develop lupus if the sibling is affected and up to 6 per cent of siblings of non-identical twins will develop lupus if the sibling is affected. And if a first degree relative (mother, father, brother or sister) has the disease, the risk is about 15 per cent. These figures compare with the general population figure of up to 0.05 per cent affected individuals. As with rheumatoid arthritis (see Chapter 6), there are a large number of genetic markers indicating lupus and its different features. There are many immune proteins, including:

▶ anti-dsDNA (involved in kidney damage in lupus)
▶ anti-RO (giving dry eye and dry mouth syndrome)
▶ anticardiolipin antibody (associated with clotting disorders and miscarriages)
▶ antiribosomal P (associated with emotional and psychiatric disturbances)
▶ antierythrocyte antibody (associated with anaemia)
▶ antiplatelet antibody (associated with bleeding disorders).

As with rheumatoid arthritis, to get lupus you must have a genetic predisposition. The specific environmental triggers are still to be discovered, but it's known that ultraviolet light and some drugs such as hydrallazine can stimulate lupus in susceptible people. So far no causes by infection have been found.

LUPUS IS ASSOCIATED WITH A RED RASH
AND SENSITIVITY TO SUNLIGHT.

INVESTIGATIONS INTO LUPUS

There are at least 58 different symptoms and signs associated with lupus and not all have to be present when you are first diagnosed, so diagnosis can be difficult. Some of the symptoms indicate lupus but may only occur in less than 1 per cent of cases. The American College of Rheumatology has listed 11 criteria for diagnosis. To confirm the diagnosis with 97 per cent accuracy, four of the following 11 criteria must be met at any time during the disease:

1 Malar rash (a red butterfly-shaped rash over the cheeks and nose).
2. Discoid rash (red raised patches of thickened skin sometimes roughly circular in shape).

3. Photosensitivity (sensitivity to sunlight, where a red rash forms on the skin in areas of the body exposed to the sun).
4. Oral ulcers on the lining of the mouth and airway at the back of the nose.
5. Arthritis affecting two or more joints.
6. Serositis (a painful inflammation of the lining of the abdominal organs, lungs and heart).
7. Renal problems (the kidneys lose essential proteins).
8. Epileptic convulsions or psychotic psychiatric symptoms.
9. Haematologic disorders (anaemia or decreased white blood cell counts).
10. Positive blood tests for anti-dsDNA or anti-Sm antibodies.
11. Positive blood test for ANA antibodies.

The diagnosis of lupus doesn't rest on any one particular test. Sometimes a blood test may be clear, but you still have all the other symptoms of the disease. I have to admit that this doesn't happen very often because in lupus so many different immune proteins are produced.

The first blood test is for ANA (anti nuclear antibody) levels, which is used as a screening test if you or your doctor suspects lupus. Ninety-five per cent of people with lupus will be positive but so will many people without lupus. ANA can be positive in the elderly without disease, in other inflammatory arthritis or a viral illness, and the use of some drugs is also known to induce ANA. Despite this, your doctor will still do this test first as it's one of the criteria for diagnosis, and more sensitive tests such as anti-dsDNA are only positive in about three-quarters of people with the disease. Anti-Sm antibodies is the most accurate blood test, but these antibodies only occur in about one-third of people.

LUPUS CAN AFFECT MANY OF YOUR ORGANS. COMMON SYMPTOMS INCLUDE FATIGUE, FEVER AND WEIGHT LOSS.

Other blood tests check for different features of the disease, such as anaemia, low white blood cells and kidney function. Urine is tested to check kidney function. Specimens collected for 24 hours can show how efficiently your kidney is operating as well as how much protein is being lost in the urine.

In general X-rays are not helpful in the investigations. Your doctor may do them to exclude other types of arthritis if a particular joint is affected. You may need specialised scans of internal organs, such as MRI, ultrasound or CT scans if your doctor thinks your brain, lung, heart or abdominal area is affected.

FEATURES OF LUPUS

Systemic lupus erythematosus starts differently in different people. In the early stage, it may affect only one organ, and others later, or it can begin full-blown. The severity of the disease also varies, ranging from mild and intermittent to persistent and severe. Most people with lupus suffer periods of flare-ups and periods of relative quietness in disease activity. A lucky 20 per cent will have remission with no further symptoms. You will probably suffer from non-specific symptoms of fatigue, fever and weight loss.

Skin

Although different types of rashes are possible, in general all of them are red. Malar, 'butterfly shaped' rashes across the cheeks and nose extending to the ears, are worse if exposed to sunlight but don't leave scars and occur in about half of sufferers. The rash often comes on suddenly and usually means your whole body (systemic) is affected. Your doctor will generally treat this with a small dose of cortisone orally and hydroxychloroquine.

About 40 per cent of people with malar rashes will lose hair (alopecia), although when the flare-up has calmed down, the hair usually regrows. If the rash spreads to other parts of your body (sub-acute cutaneous lupus) it's also non-scarring, photosensitive and indicates disease activity and arthritis. You will also feel tired.

Discoid lupus erythematosus produces roundish rashes with a raised edge, scaliness and associated small skin veins. The rashes are photosensitive and can occur virtually anywhere on the body. If you have symptoms like this, you may also experience permanent hair loss, loss of skin pigment and scarring. Your doctor will usually treat this with cortisone creams and ointments applied to the rash, or cortisone injected into the rash. If you have a rash like this, avoid exposure to sunlight by wearing long sleeves and pants.

Like all the developments of lupus, the rashes are a direct result of immune proteins being deposited in the blood vessels. If these immune protein complexes end up in the blood vessels of the kidney, kidney damage results—this is also true for other organs. Because there are so many different types of immune proteins being produced, there are an infinite number of ways you can experience lupus.

IF YOU HAVE A RASH ASSOCIATED WITH LUPUS, WEAR LONG SLEEVES AND PANTS, TO MINIMISE YOUR EXPOSURE TO SUNLIGHT.

Joints and muscles

About 95 per cent of people who develop lupus will experience aches and pains in the joints and muscles but this doesn't necessarily mean you'll develop arthritis. If you're one of the 60 per cent who does develop arthritis, it often only lasts a short time, although it may be recurrent. The joints affected are usually the knuckles, the finger joints nearest the knuckles, wrists and knees. The joints are often quite swollen and there might be associated inflammation of the synovium of the tendons. Fortunately joint deformities in the hands are uncommon. If deformities do form they may be similar to the deformities of rheumatoid arthritis. You may also get lupus nodules of the skin, which look similar to rheumatoid nodules but which develop differently.

When lupus is active, your muscles can become inflamed resulting in myositis, or muscle breakdown. This occurs in 40 per cent of people. Some of the treatments for lupus, such as cortisone, can also induce muscle wasting and osteoporosis. The bone blood supply may also die off (ischaemic necrosis) and causes pain in the bones. This happens in 15 per cent of cases. The cause of bone ischaemic necrosis is due to immune proteins associated with lupus floating around in the blood and eventually depositing in the artery wall, setting off inflammation within the blood vessel (vasculitis). The vessel becomes so inflamed that the blood supply to the bone is stopped and that part of the bone dies.

Kidneys

The proteins of the immune system, produced in the blood in lupus, tend to deposit themselves out of the blood vessels and into kidney tissue. The proteins stimulate inflammation of the kidney and if this isn't treated the kidney will eventually be destroyed (lupus-induced glomerulonephritis). If the kidneys aren't working properly, large amounts of protein are lost in the urine and you may become protein deficient, as well as suffer fluid retention with associated ankle, leg, hand and facial swelling.

If the kidneys become severely affected, you can develop kidney failure and may need life support with renal dialysis or kidney transplantation. Kidney failure may happen slowly and insidiously or rapidly and aggressively.

Because of the life-threatening consequences, severe disease needs strong treatment with high doses of cortisone and toxic immunosuppressives such as azathioprine or cyclophosphamide. If you have persistent protein in the urine or high levels of anti-dsDNA, you're at risk of developing severe kidney disease. You may need a renal biopsy, which can show the outlook and severity of kidney damage. This is done by looking at the microscopic location of the deposited immune protein complexes, the type of cell damage and how active and chronic the damage to the kidney is. Although up to half of people with lupus can develop significant loss of protein in the urine, only 5 to 10 per cent of these are at risk of developing life-threatening kidney failure.

Nervous system

Lupus affects the brain, spinal cord or nerves in about 60 per cent of cases. Usually the nervous system is only affected if other major organs are affected at the same time; you can either get a single or cluster of symptoms. One of the most common symptoms is memory loss and the feeling that you're not able to think straight. This affects half of lupus sufferers, but fortunately is usually mild. Headaches, sometimes severe, are also common. Some people also have epileptic seizures. Because the brain has many different functions the symptoms can be diverse. Less frequent possibilities include:

▶ psychosis (hearing voices and hallucinating)
▶ coordination problems
▶ diabetes insipidus (increased thirst and urination)
▶ visual loss if the retina or visual part of the brain is affected
▶ bleeding around the brain
▶ strokes
▶ nerves not working properly in the legs and arms.

It's difficult to conclusively establish whether your lupus is affecting the nervous system, so the suspicion factor will always play a role in diagnosis.

Although electroencephalograms are positive in many people, that only confirms the diagnosis of a convulsion and doesn't necessarily show that lupus is the cause. Findings from high-tech scans like CT and MRI are non-specific. Even putting a needle in the spine and taking spinal fluid for investigation doesn't confirm the diagnosis of lupus affecting the nervous system, although it will help exclude other possibilities such as infection and multiple sclerosis.

A COMMON SYMPTOM OF LUPUS IS LOSS OF MEMORY OR FREQUENT HEADACHES. OF COURSE, NOT ALL HEADACHES OR LAPSES OF MEMORY MEAN YOU HAVE THE DISEASE.

Blood vessels

There are two ways blood vessels can be damaged by lupus. First, they can be hit with inflammation, which leads to the swelling of the vessel and eventual blockage. The consequence of this is a loss of blood supply to the surrounding tissues, which then die. If the heart is affected you could have a heart attack; if the brain is affected you could have a stroke; and if the kidney is affected you could have kidney failure. The amount of damage depends on how big the blood vessel is and how much tissue is supplied by that vessel.

DAMAGED BLOOD VESSELS CAN LEAD TO THE RISK OF HEART ATTACK, STROKE OR KIDNEY FAILURE.

The second way lupus damages blood vessels is by its ability to induce thrombosis (in about 15 per cent of cases). Thrombosis is clotting of the blood within a vein or artery, which means there is loss of blood supply to the tissues. If a vein is affected, more commonly the clot could break off and return to the heart and lungs, inducing the potentially life-threatening condition 'pulmonary embolus' if the clot is big enough. Fortunately, the risk of thrombosis in lupus is easy to confirm by a blood test for anticardiolipin antibody. If this is positive, you will need to use a lifelong anti-coagulant medication.

Bone marrow and blood

If your lupus is active, you'll probably be one of approximately two-thirds of people who become anaemic. Your body's resources are being used to combat the disease, and so there's little left over to produce new red blood cells. When disease activity recedes, the anaemia improves. The immune system's white blood cells may also decrease, but this is usually mild and an increased risk of infections is rare. The platelets (small cells) of the blood are susceptible to lupus, which affects their production in the bone marrow. If the platelet count becomes very low, spontaneous bleeding can occur. You will need a quick and aggressive treatment for the lupus in order to switch off this tendency.

Heart and lungs

Sixty per cent of lupus patients will develop heart or lung problems, but of these only 10 per cent will be serious. The most common problem is inflammation of the linings of the heart or lung, leading to either pericarditis (heart) or a form of pleurisy (lung). Although both conditions can be painful, they don't usually have serious consequences and are often relieved by aspirin or other non-steroidals.

Inflammation of the heart muscle (myocarditis) can result in heart failure, abnormal heart rhythms and, rarely, sudden death. About 10 per cent of people with lupus have myocarditis. If the lining of your heart chambers becomes inflamed, the heart valves can be damaged, which can lead to either a blockage of outflow from the chamber or a back-flow of blood back into the chamber (especially if the valve doesn't close properly). This strains your heart and eventually leads to heart failure. Heart valve damage occurs in a small number of people, and if the valve damage is bad enough you may need a valve replacement.

You may also get pleurisy, in which fluid collects around the lungs and means the lung can't expand properly within the chest until the fluid is removed, either naturally by your body, or with a needle by your doctor. Shortness of breath is a common symptom. Inflammation of the actual lung tissue occurs in only about 10 per cent of people with lupus. You will need aggressive treatment because if it persists, the lung tissue can become scarred. This is permanent and non-treatable, and you'll look and feel like someone suffering from emphysema. If you have lupus, you'll be at increased risk of lung infection and you should see you doctor urgently if you have symptoms of cough, shortness of breath and fever. It's also a good idea to get yearly immunisations for influenza and 10-yearly immunisations for *streptococcus pneumonia*, which is the most common cause of pneumonia.

*IF YOU EXPERIENCE COUGHS, SHORTNESS OF BREATH
OR FEVER, SEE YOUR DOCTOR IMMEDIATELY, AS THESE
SYMPTOMS MAY INDICATE A LUNG INFECTION.*

A very small number of people with lupus get a fatal complication, alveolar haemorrhage, in which the blood vessels of the lung become so inflamed that they rupture, causing severe bleeding into the air sacs of the lung. The lungs fill with blood, and unless you're treated promptly, you could die.

The abdomen

There are many organs in the abdomen that can be affected by lupus. Forty per cent of people experience liver abnormalities, but these aren't severe and usually return to normal once the disease has been treated or goes into a quiet phase. Abdominally related symptoms of loss of appetite, nausea, mild pain and diarrhoea are common. In some people with lupus, vasculitis can affect the blood vessels supplying the bowel—if that part of the bowel dies from lack of blood supply, you can get bowel perforation and peritonitis. Emergency surgery and intravenous antibiotics are the only answer to this problem. If the pancreas becomes inflamed, you'll experience severe abdominal pain. This can also be life-threatening, and needs emergency treatment in hospital.

*SEVERE ABDOMINAL PAIN MAY INDICATE
AN INFLAMED ORGAN FROM LUPUS.*

The eyes

A small number of people (about 5 per cent) with lupus can develop vasculitis affecting the blood vessels of the retina. This needs immediate treatment, as you could quickly go blind within a few days. Other eye complications include inflammation of the conjunctiva and the white of the eyes (scleritis) and damage to the optic nerve. The lacrimal gland, which produces tears, can also be damaged which will make your eyes dry, scratchy and inflamed.

Drug-induced systemic lupus erythematosus

Some people, especially those with slow-acting livers who have a genetic disposition, can develop lupus from certain drugs. The most common drugs to cause lupus-like symptoms are procainamide (used for abnormal heart rhythms) and hydrallazine (used for severe blood pressure), although it's rare for these drugs to be prescribed. Lupus-like reactions with other drugs are extremely rare but can happen with penicillamine, chlorpromazine, methyldopa, quinidine, interferon alpha and possibly the oral contraceptive pill.

Common effects of the drugs include arthritis, pleurisy, pericarditis and various effects on the bone marrow. The treatment for drug-induced lupus is simple and usually means stopping the drug. A small number of people affected may need a short course of cortisone to settle the complaint. It's unusual for symptoms to last longer than six months. Surprisingly, these drugs can safely be given to people with true lupus.

Pregnancy
Fertility rates are normal in lupus and if there are no severe renal or heart problems and the disease is controlled, your pregnancy will go to term with the delivery of a normal baby. In a small percentage of pregnant women lupus can flare-up during pregnancy and during the six weeks after birth. Rarely, the baby is affected by the mother's lupus and can have heart abnormalities or low platelet counts.

FERTILITY RATES ARE NORMAL IN LUPUS AND IF THE DISEASE IS CONTROLLED, THERE IS NO REASON WHY YOU WON'T DELIVER A FULL-TERM, HEALTHY BABY.

Although you still have a normal ability to fall pregnant, there is an increased risk of miscarriage or stillbirth. It especially occurs in women who have anti-cardiolipin antibodies in the blood, which cause thrombosis (blood clots). Treatments aimed at stopping these two complications in lupus are still controversial and may include blood-thinning medications throughout the pregnancy.

TREATMENT OF LUPUS
Treatment options depend on how severe the lupus is and what symptoms you have. You will usually be given narcotic-based pain killers, such as codeine for pain, although it's better to use paracetamol. Arthritis-type pain, pleurisy and pericarditis pain respond to non-steroidal anti-

inflammatory medications. Hydroxychloroquinine is one of the few disease-modifying agents that effectively treats the arthritis of lupus.

You can use small doses of cortisone-based medications to improve symptoms of malaise, lethargy and chronic tiredness. Lupus may make you so lethargic that you have trouble getting out of bed. Cortisone will relieve this and you can start enjoying life again. It will also help relieve the aching pain from lupus arthritis. You and your doctor can weigh up the side effects of cortisone medications against your quality of life without it.

Hydroxychloroquine can settle a lupus rash within a few weeks. Using maximum-rating sun screens, or better still, avoiding the sun altogether, are the best courses of action with photosensitive rashes.

Severe lupus needs radical treatment, otherwise you will get severe organ damage or failure. The usual treatment is high dose cortisone, either orally or intravenously. As your situation stabilises, your doctor will gradually decrease the cortisone dose until the minimal dose to achieve disease control is found. This dose is variable so you'll need close monitoring. If long-term cortisone treatment is the only alternative, you'll need to counteract the side effects. Where possible, take osteoporosis-preventing medications—if you're post-menopausal you should have oestrogen supplements if you're able to take them. High blood pressure needs to be controlled fastidiously to preserve kidney function and if you have a risk of high blood sugar you'll need to modify your diet.

As a last resort you can take either cyclophosphamide or azathioprine in combination with cortisone. These combinations have been found to decrease flare-ups of lupus and to decrease the development of kidney failure. They don't decrease mortality rates but do improve quality of life. The potentially serious side effects (see Chapter 2, Disease-modifying drugs) need close monitoring by your doctor but the advantage of using these drugs is that a smaller dose of cortisone is used, so there's a decreased risk of cortisone-related side effects.

Some features of lupus don't respond to cortisone, cyclophosphamide or azathioprine. Clotting disorders need thinning of the blood with either Warfarin orally, or Heparin by injections. Lupus can affect the frontal lobe of the brain, inducing behavioural disturbances and if this happens, you'll be given medication to stop the hallucinations.

WHAT TO EXPECT

There is no cure for lupus. Two years after diagnosis, the survival rate is about 95 per cent. At five years, the survival rate is about 90 per cent, at 10 years 75 per cent and at 20 years 70 per cent. A poor outlook is more likely if there is significant kidney involvement, high blood pressure, anaemia and serious nervous system involvement. The most common causes of fatalities associated with lupus are secondary infections and kidney failure in the early stages and blood clotting problems later on in the disease. Other significant factors include low socioeconomic status and a non-Caucasian background. Disability is common with lupus and often lethargy, pain and fatigue are major problems. Twenty per cent of people with lupus will have remissions lasting up to five years and half of these remissions may last for decades. Approximately one-quarter of lupus sufferers will have mild disease without any life-threatening consequences.

SCLERODERMA

Hardening of the skin—scleroderma—is one of the more obvious features of this disease. Skin hardening which is called fibrosis, happens at the end of the inflammation process when normal tissue is replaced by scar tissue. Like other forms of inflammatory arthritis, scleroderma doesn't just affect joints and skin—other organ involvement, including lung, gut, heart, blood vessels and muscles, is more critical. Sometimes scleroderma can also affect the internal organs without affecting the skin.

There are two main forms of scleroderma. Diffuse scleroderma affecting the skin of the arms, legs, torso and face is distributed symmetrically between the two sides of the body. It usually starts quickly with other organs, such as the heart and lung, being affected early in the disease. Limited scleroderma, on the other hand, still affects the skin symmetrically but is slower in its progression and doesn't tend to affect other organs. A variant of limited scleroderma, CREST, stands for:

▶ Calcinosis (calcium deposits around joints and in soft tissue)
▶ Raynaud's phenomenon (severe colour changes to the hands and feet associated with cold skin)
▶ Esophageal dismotility (heartburn and acid reflux into the gullet and mouth)
▶ Sclerodactyly (hardened, stiff fingers and toes)
▶ Telangectasia (small veins forming on the body, hands and face).

The long-term outlook for limited scleroderma is much better than for diffuse scleroderma.

STATISTICS AND CAUSES OF SCLERODERMA

Scleroderma rarely affects children or young men—women are three times more likely to get the disease than men—and its initial presentation is usually between the ages of 20 and 40 years. There appears to be a hereditary tendency, but like some other forms of arthritis, it needs an environmental trigger.

Environmental factors

Coal and gold miners have an increased risk of developing the disease because of their exposure to silica dust. Polyvinyl chloride (PVC) production workers are also at risk of developing some skin features of scleroderma and rarely may also develop liver cirrhosis and cancers of blood vessels. Benzene and toluene production is also associated with development of the disease. In Spain, 20,000 people developed a scleroderma-like condition involving lungs, joints, muscles and skin, which was supposedly caused by a particular rapeseed cooking oil. Scleroderma symptoms can also be induced by certain drugs, such as bleomycin (used in cancer) and pentazocine (a pain killer), but these are not widely used.

THE NATURE OF THE DISEASE

The protein collagen, produced by skin cells (fibroblasts), gives the skin its structural strength and shape. Fibroblasts and collagen are also present in other organs in the body. The major problem with scleroderma is an over-production of collagen associated with an over-stimulation of fibroblast activity. The immune system is also over-stimulated, causing extensive blood vessel damage, and this is the basis of the disease.

Blood vessel injury, an early feature of scleroderma, leads to the development of Raynaud's phenomenon—a decreased blood flow to the fingers and toes. It seems to prefer the small blood vessels and, as well as affecting the digits, it damages the small blood vessels of internal organs. When blood vessels are inflamed they swell and thicken, and blood flow diminishes. Eventually the blood vessel is totally obliterated and surrounding vessels may swell up to take the extra blood flow, resulting in small swollen veins of the skin (telangectasia).

WHEN THE IMMUNE SYSTEM IS OVER-STIMULATED, TOO MUCH COLLAGEN IS PRODUCED AND EXTENSIVE BLOOD VESSEL DAMAGE RESULTS.

Damage to the blood vessels is caused by an overproduction of immune proteins that stimulate inflammation. When this happens, the blood vessel cells release other proteins, which then act to stimulate the fibroblasts to overproduce collagen. The stimulated fibroblasts can produce two to three times the normal amount of collagen and this goes on indefinitely. The stimulated fibroblasts release other proteins, which then stimulate the immune cells to release even more fibroblast-stimulating proteins, and a vicious circle develops. The damaged tissue is replaced with new scar-like tissue that's not able to function as normal tissue. If an internal organ is affected by this process the efficiency of that organ is compromised. If, eventually, the organ is replaced by fibrotic scar tissue, organ failure can result. In people without scleroderma, fibroblast proteins and immune cell proteins have a switching off mechanism that stops the collagen production once enough is produced. If you have scleroderma you have lost that regulatory mechanism and collagen production goes haywire.

FEATURES OF SCLERODERMA

The diagnosis of scleroderma is straightforward if you have classic changes of the skin and a major organ is involved. Initially it may look like you have rheumatoid arthritis, systemic lupus erythematosus or polymyositis but as the skin becomes affected the diagnosis is confirmed.

Skin

Almost everyone with scleroderma has skin problems. Typically the skin of the hands and fingers becomes swollen and tight. It may progress to the arms, legs and face, where the skin gradually thickens and becomes firm. The inflammation of this process leads to scarring under the skin until the skin becomes firmly bound to the underlying tissue. Beginning on the extremities, the condition advances up the limbs and eventually the torso. These changes develop over several months to years.

THE SKIN EVENTUALLY TAKES ON A SMOOTH, SHINY QUALITY.

If the skin changes occur rapidly over a two-year period your internal organs are also probably affected, especially the lungs, heart and kidneys. In limited scleroderma, the skin changes are usually restricted to the fingers and toes with only slow progression of further skin changes affecting other parts of your skin. The skin changes usually happen over a period of five years and then might gradually improve. After many years, your skin may return to normal and soften, or become thin and worn. If the skin softens, it does it in the reverse order to how it started, usually with the softening beginning on your trunk and ending on the extremities of the fingers and toes.

As the skin tightens on the fingers, it will become harder to bend your finger joints and the joints may become permanently bent. This is called a contracture. If the blood vessels are inflamed and the skin is especially tight, the blood supply may be cut off and the skin may die, forming an ulcer. This may happen on the pads of the fingers and over bony prominences such as the elbows and ankles. Blood supply to the bone may also stop and the bone of the fingertips disappears.

Skin pigment can either increase or decrease and the fibrosis of the skin destroys hair follicles leading to hair loss. Sweat glands are also lost, drying the skin into coarseness.

THE LOSS OF SKIN WRINKLES, TIGHTNESS AROUND THE MOUTH, AND A POINTY NOSE ARE DISTINCTIVE FEATURES OF SCLERODERMA.

Raynaud's phenomenon
If you have scleroderma, there's a 95 per cent chance you have Raynaud's phenomenon, although some people without scleroderma also have it.

Cold weather, smoking and other types of inflammatory arthritis can bring on Raynaud's phenomenon.

Caused by inflammation and irritation of small arteries in the skin, this in turn leads to contraction of the muscular coating of these arteries. The result is a smaller diameter to the blood vessel and a markedly decreased blood flow to the skin. Your skin will be cold and can become white, red or blue depending on the amount of blood getting through. You might have associated pins and needles and pain if the skin's nerves lose their blood supply. Raynaud's phenomenon especially affects the fingers and toes, but can also affect the nose and ears. You could have these changes several years before the skin changes of scleroderma. But if you have diffuse scleroderma, skin changes may only take several months to develop.

Joints and muscles

If you have scleroderma, you have a 70 per cent chance of developing pain, swelling and stiffness of the joints, particularly the fingers and knees. In early stages the arthritis features will resemble rheumatoid arthritis but as scleroderma develops it will take on its own feature of creaking and cracking of the joint, much like the sound of old leather being bent.

Muscle weakness is common, because when the disease is active, the muscles aren't being used. With treatment this weakness is reversed. About 5 per cent of people develop an inflammation of a muscle of the upper legs or arms resulting in permanent damage.

The gut

The oesophagus or gullet is the main site in the gut for scleroderma. Acid from the stomach regurgitates into the oesophagus and burns its lining, often resulting in ulceration. Common symptoms include a burning pain in the pit of the stomach extending into the chest, the feeling of food becoming stuck in mid-chest after swallowing, and acid refluxing into the back of the throat.

Your oesophagus could be affected in three ways. The fibrotic scarring can damage the muscles of the oesophagus so they don't efficiently push food downwards and it feels as if the food is stuck. Secondly, there is a muscular ring between the oesophagus and the stomach which, when it contracts, acts as a physical barrier between the two. This is a protective mechanism to stop the reflux of acid from the stomach into the gullet, as the lining of the stomach has been designed to tolerate acid while the oesophageal lining has not. If this muscle ring is damaged, acid splashes into the oesophagus and burns it. Thirdly, a combination of muscle damage and acid exposure to the gullet may lead to severe scarring and a stricture may form, making the passage of food down the oesophagus even harder.

Lastly, oesophageal function can be affected by damage to its nerve supply. If the nerves are damaged by scleroderma the muscles won't be able to contract in a coordinated way to help the passage of food and existing symptoms of an oesophagus affected by scleroderma will be worsened.

THE FEELING OF FOOD BECOMING STUCK IN THE CHEST AND ACID REFLUX INTO THE BACK OF THE THROAT ARE SIGNS THAT THE OESOPHAGUS MAY BE AFFECTED BY SCLERODERMA.

Rarely, the intestines and large bowel can also be affected by scleroderma. If your intestinal muscles are affected, inefficient movement of bowel contents results, often leading to abdominal bloating, wind colic, constipation and even bowel obstruction. If you experience diarrhoea and weight loss, it's due to a secondary overgrowth of bowel bacteria caused by inefficient movement of the bowel contents. A few people can have severe bleeding from the bowel because of the formation of telangectasia (swollen veins) in the bowel lining, the same as they form in the skin. As these small veins are under a greater amount of pressure there's the possibility that they can rupture and haemorrhage into the bowel.

The lungs

Progressive shortness of breath with an associated dry, non-productive cough could mean your lungs are affected. It's important to see your doctor straight away as this complication could be fatal. The damage done to lung tissue makes it highly susceptible to infections and pneumonia can be a serious complication. If you have severe reflux, you can inhale stomach acid into the lungs when asleep, often resulting in pneumonia.

The major damage to the lungs in scleroderma is to the small air sacs, the alveoli. These sacs are delicate membranes that allow the passage of gases into and out of the blood. In scleroderma, they are susceptible to damage and easily become scarred. When the alveoli is scarred it becomes fibrotic and its ability to allow oxygen transfer into the blood and carbon dioxide out of the blood is virtually zero. This means the body can't get enough oxygen for its needs and can't effectively remove waste products (carbon dioxide). The blood vessels that run next to the alveoli that pick up oxygen from the lung and take it back to the heart and the rest of the body are also affected by the fibrotic scarring and blood can't flow through them. This puts a strain on the heart as it's trying to pump blood through damaged and obliterated blood vessels. Heart failure can result, although fortunately this doesn't happen in most patients.

SHORTNESS OF BREATH AND A DRY COUGH MAY INDICATE THAT THE LUNGS ARE AFFECTED BY SCLERODERMA.

The heart
Most people with diffuse scleroderma have some form of heart problem. The pericardium (the sac around the heart) may be affected, resulting in an accumulation of fluid around the heart, which can make it harder for the heart to pump blood around the body. Scleroderma can affect the electrical conduction network in the heart giving abnormal heart rhythms that can occasionally be life-threatening or it can damage the heart muscle leading to a cardiomyopathy and heart failure. Cardiomyopathy affects less than 10 per cent of individuals with scleroderma.

Kidneys
People with rapidly developing skin thickening during the first two to three years of diffuse scleroderma have a high risk of kidney disease (although people with other forms of scleroderma are not at risk). Renal crisis is characterised by very high blood pressure, which rapidly initiates kidney failure. For this reason it's important you control your blood pressure.

Other features
Scleroderma does have some other features in common with other types of inflammatory arthritis. Probably the most common is Sjogren's syndrome (see Chapter 11), with symptoms including an irritating dry mouth and dry eyes. Using frequent mouth washes and nutrient drops for the eyes helps this situation, which is caused by the destruction of the salivary glands and the destruction of the lacrimal glands that produce the nutrient-containing tears.

Other features of scleroderma are uncommon. Your face and tongue may feel numb and painful. This is caused by damage to the trigeminal nerves which supply sensation to the face and part of the taste nerve supply. Hypothyroidism, in which the thyroid gland in the neck is attacked and becomes under-active, can also occur. The thyroid is essential in the control of metabolism, and underactivity leads to tiredness and a general slowness of functioning of the body's vital organs. If untreated it can lead to slowing of the heart and brain. In men, impotence can be because of vascular damage to the penis and damage to its nerve supply. A small number of people can develop liver cirrhosis.

INVESTIGATIONS INTO SCLERODERMA

Initial investigations include a full blood count (FBC) that usually shows an anaemia secondary to chronic disease activity. The erythrocyte sedimentation rate (ESR) will usually be elevated to indicate how active the disease is. Another indicator is the immune protein anti-topoisomerase 1 antibody, which is very specific for scleroderma but is only positive in 40 per cent of cases. Anticentromere antibody is positive in up to 80 per cent of people with CREST form of scleroderma. Anti-RNA polymerase antibodies I, II & III are found in diffuse scleroderma and often show a high risk of renal and cardiac problems.

Investigations after the diagnosis is confirmed are for monitoring the disease and its progress. Your doctor may order lung function tests to measure lung volumes and how well oxygen is being transferred to blood from the alveoli. Chest X-rays look for other causes of lung deterioration and lung CT scans look for inflammation of the lung tissue. Ultrasounds of the heart look for structural problems with the heart valves and also determine how well the heart is performing. Ultrasounds of the kidneys look at structural aspects and 24-hour collections of urine examine kidney function. Blood tests can determine kidney function, but the 24-hour urine test is more sensitive. If you have oesophagal symptoms, you may also need examination by a fibre-optic endoscope (a high-tech telescope with a miniature camera) to check the extent of damage to the lining of the oesophagus.

TREATMENTS FOR SCLERODERMA

As scleroderma is uncommon, many treatments are still to be fully researched. It's difficult to gather enough people with scleroderma to give a research study statistical significance, but there are sufficient anecdotal cases in the medical literature to show which drugs work and which ones don't.

Diffuse scleroderma is a potentially fatal disease so needs an aggressive treatment approach, especially if the kidney, heart or lungs are affected. Initially you will need to take cortisone and a disease-modifying drug. Some of the disease modifiers don't have any effect on scleroderma, but the use of penicillamine, azathioprine, cyclophosphamide, methotrexate and 5-flurouracil (an anti-cancer agent) have been shown to slow the progress of the disease in some people. Other drugs such as cyclosporin and gamma-interferon may also be of help although they are very expensive and are not widely used.

The choice of drug depends on how severe your illness is and which organs are affected. Your doctor will also be looking at possible side effects and whether there is any kidney failure as this determines blood levels of the drug. Cortisone is generally used initially to stop collections of fluid developing around the heart and to stop muscle involvement. Once these conditions have settled, the dose can be slowly decreased and eventually withdrawn if possible. You can take cortisone daily or in large pulse doses weekly to monthly. Low doses of cortisone have been shown to slow the degree of lung damage.

Other drugs are used to modify symptoms. Drugs such as penicillamine, vitamin E and captopril have been shown in some people to soften the skin changes. Penicillamine is used as a disease modifier—it also breaks down collagen bonds in the skin so that your skin doesn't become scarred and stick to its underlying layers. Captopril, as well as helping with skin softening, helps to preserve kidney function by minimising pressures around the kidney cells.

Symptoms associated with the oesophagus can often be improved with drugs that decrease the stomach's acid production. These drugs include omeprazole, ranitidine and famotidine and are frequently used to treat peptic ulcers. Cisapride works by increasing stomach emptying, which means there is less to reflux into the oesophagus. This drug is less popular as it can lead to potentially dangerous heart rhythms. Elevating the head of the bed lessens the effect of gravity when lying down—a supine position increases acid reflux into the oesophagus.

The arthritis that develops with scleroderma often responds to non-steroidal anti-inflammatory medications. If you're one of the small proportion of people who don't respond to these drugs, low-dose cortisone may help your painful joints.

Treatments for Raynaud's phenomenon don't always work, and even when they do, they are usually unable to be tolerated in the long term. Recommended drugs include nifedipine, diltiazem, nitrates, prazosin and alphamethyldopa. If you have a very bad case of Raynaud's phenomenon you can try injections of local anaesthetic or chemicals into the nerves in the neck which switch off the blood vessel nerves and relieve symptoms. You need to repeat these injections, but again they're not always successful.

Complications of scleroderma such as heart failure and high blood pressure can be treated by the usual appropriate medications for these conditions.

WHAT TO EXPECT

Because vital organs are involved with diffuse scleroderma, it is potentially more serious than limited scleroderma where you can expect to live for over 20 years from time of diagnosis. However renal dialysis and kidney and lung transplants have improved the outlook for those suffering from diffuse scleroderma. Sixty per cent of people can now expect to live 10 years, although the prognosis can be poorer for older men.

CHAPTER | 10

SARCOIDOSIS

S arcoidosis is another inflammatory disease that can affect joints and many other organs in the body, especially the lung, followed by lymph nodes, skin and the eyes.

The disease often occurs suddenly and for many people it becomes chronic, coming and going over several years.

STATISTICS AND CAUSES OF SARCOIDOSIS

As for most chronic inflammatory arthritic conditions, the exact cause of sarcoidosis is unknown. Although a number of infections are suspected of inducing the disease, there is not enough convincing evidence to yet reach a conclusion. Like other forms of arthritis you need to have a genetic predisposition and the disease must be triggered by an infection or something else in the environment. There have been cases of sarcoidosis in families and also in husband and wife pairs. Some communities of unrelated people in a geographic area also have been affected, suggesting local environmental influences. No particular genetic markers have been found for sarcoidosis and sarcoidosis affecting the lung has actually been found to afflict non-smokers to a greater degree than smokers.

Sarcoidosis is one of the more common inflammatory diseases and affects all races. An equal number of men and women across all ages can get the disease, but it usually develops in the 20 to 40 year age group.

THE NATURE OF THE DISEASE

When sarcoidosis starts, white blood cells (phagocytes) gather within the tissue of the affected organ or joint. Phagocytes are immune cells often referred to as the scavengers of the human body. If you have bacteria, a damaged cell or a foreign body inside you, the phagocyte will surround and ingest it so that it's cleaned up and removed from your body. As the disease progresses, the phagocytes aggregate to form small granules or nodules within the affected tissue (granulomas).

As long as the tissue doesn't become inflamed, the granuloma is considered to be harmless to the surrounding tissue. But the tissue architecture can become distorted. For example, in the lung, the bulk of the granuloma compresses the airways and blood vessels resulting in decreased lung volumes and shortness of breath. When the disease is suppressed or goes into spontaneous remission, the number of granulomas decreases, the distortion of the organ tissue tends to return to normal and your symptoms disappear. If the tissue is inflamed for a long period of time, fibrosis and scarring of the tissue can result even if the sarcoidosis goes away. Occasionally, the scarred areas remain permanently damaged and your organs could fail.

FEATURES OF SARCOIDOSIS

Sarcoidosis can be generalised or restricted to one organ, but the lung is nearly always affected. The disease usually starts abruptly over a week or so, but it can also develop over several months. Occasionally your doctor may find sarcoidosis when doing routine checks for other problems.

Fever, malaise, weight loss and loss of appetite are the usual initial symptoms. There are often lung-associated symptoms, such as a dry cough, shortness of breath and chest discomfort. The accompanying arthritis often affects more than four joints at the one time. Your salivary gland may also get bigger, your eyes inflamed, nerves may become paralysed.

SARCOIDOSIS IS OFTEN ACCIDENTALLY
DETECTED ON A CHEST X-RAY.

The lungs

If your doctor suspects sarcoidosis, he or she will probably refer you for a chest X-ray. For most people, the X-ray shows some abnormality. About half the people who get sarcoidosis will develop permanent abnormalities of the lung, but usually this is mild. The inflammation of lung tissue in sarcoidosis affects the main areas of gas exchange between the lungs and blood—the air sacs (alveoli) and the blood vessels of the lung.

Occasionally the lymph node around the bronchi (the main tubes of the lung) enlarges and compresses the bronchi, making it more difficult for you to breathe. Inflammation of the lining of the lung means fluid can accumulate in the chest cavity—you will need to have this drained.

A DRY COUGH, SHORTNESS OF BREATH AND
SOME CHEST DISCOMFORT MAY SUGGEST THAT
YOUR LUNGS ARE AFFECTED.

Lymph nodes

Enlargement of lymph nodes is very common in sarcoidosis, especially the nodes within the chest cavity. Lymph node enlargement also occurs in the neck, armpit and groin. These enlargements are not a big problem, unless they become large enough to be disfiguring or if they compress other organs and so interfere with their functioning.

Skin

A common problem in sarcoidosis is the development of tender, red nodules (erythema nodosum) on the shins if a joint is also affected or if the disease is flaring up. Other rashes, plaques and eruptions can affect the skin in sarcoidosis but these aren't as frequent.

The eyes

About one-quarter of people with sarcoidosis suffer an inflammation of the iris and surrounding structures. If this isn't treated by cortisone it can lead to blindness. If you have blurred vision, a watery eye and a sensitivity to bright light, ask your doctor to make the appropriate tests. Other parts of the eye that can be affected are the conjunctiva, leading to conjunctivitis, and the tear gland, which dries up tear production leading to a dry-eye syndrome of irritable, scratchy eyes.

WATERY EYES AND BLURRED VISION CAN SOMETIMES BE THE RESULT OF AN INFLAMMATION OF THE IRIS. SEE YOUR DOCTOR IF YOU HAVE THESE SYMPTOMS.

Mouth, nose and throat

The lining of the nose can become inflamed and you may also find your nose is stuffy and blocked. The tonsils can become enlarged and sarcoidosis can affect the larynx leading to obstruction of breathing. If this happens you need urgent surgery to stop you from suffocating.

Bone marrow

In about 40 per cent of cases the bone marrow is affected. However the symptoms are only mild – you may have slight anaemia, a small increase in immune white cell count and your spleen may become enlarged, but this gives minimal side effects.

The liver and kidneys

Although many people with this disease will get an enlarged liver, this is rarely a medical problem. The kidneys are rarely damaged, but the sarcoidosis can induce high levels of calcium in the blood. The calcium is deposited in the kidney and forms kidney stones.

Joints

About half the people with sarcoidosis get arthritis, which mostly occurs in the large joints like the hips, knees and shoulders. Although it generally doesn't spread, a few people can develop joint destruction or deformities. Bone cysts due to sarcoidosis are rare.

The heart

If a sarcoid lesion affects the electrical network of the heart, you may experience heart rhythm problems or, occasionally, heart failure, inflammation of the sac around the heart and heart valve lesions.

The nervous system

Only a few people will have brain, spinal cord and nerve problems. The facial nerve is most commonly affected, resulting in a short-term facial paralysis. If the optic nerve is affected you may have some loss of vision, and if the nerve to the ear is affected you could become deaf. Convulsions to the brain can sometimes occur.

The hormonal system

If the pituitary gland at the base of the brain becomes inflamed with sarcoidosis, it can result in diabetes insipidus (not related to sugar diabetes). This condition makes you very thirsty and you'll urinate more often due to a lack of anti-diuretic hormone. The adrenal glands can be affected resulting in a decreased production of natural cortisone. Pregnancy improves sarcoidosis although you could have flare-ups after the baby is born.

IF THE PITUITARY GLAND IS AFFECTED, YOU MAY BECOME VERY THIRSTY AND NEED TO URINATE FREQUENTLY.

INVESTIGATIONS INTO SARCOIDOSIS

There are no specific initial investigations for sarcoidosis, and your doctor will use tests to exclude other diseases. Chest X-rays often show enlarged lymph nodes around the large airways of the lungs. If the lungs are affected badly, they will be fibrous and scarred. Sometimes nodules of granuloma material may also show up on the X-ray.

A lung biopsy is the only way to diagnose sarcoidosis with accuracy. This is usually done via a fibre-optic telescope with a camera, which is passed down into the bronchi of the lung through the mouth. It's a safe procedure but in some difficult cases a lung biopsy with a needle guided by X-ray control may be necessary to sample affected tissue.

A LUNG BIOPSY IS DONE USING A FIBRE-OPTIC TELESCOPE WHICH IS PASSED THROUGH THE MOUTH AND INTO THE BRONCHI OF THE LUNGS.

To monitor the disease and responses to treatment, it's important your doctor does lung function tests. These tests measure the lung volumes and ability of oxygen to cross into the blood from the air sacs. In sarcoidosis the volume of your lungs is decreased so the lungs transfer less oxygen to the blood.

There is no specific blood test to diagnose this disease but a blood test to monitor the disease—angiotensin converting enzyme—which goes up and down depending on disease activity. This test is usually only used once the diagnosis has been confirmed on biopsy as it also becomes raised in some other diseases.

TREATMENT OF SARCOIDOSIS

Cortisone is the most successful treatment but because of the significant side effects with long-term use, you should only take it if benefits outweigh the risks. The main criteria for using cortisone are:

▶ disabling symptoms such as fever, shortness of breath or arthritis
▶ malfunction of organs such as of the lungs, eyes, heart or nervous system
▶ enlarged lymph nodes, which lead to significant organ distortion and malfunction.

If you start on a course of cortisone, you'll probably be on it for at least 12 months. Your doctor will reduce the starting dose over several months to try to minimise side effects. There is some anecdotal evidence to suggest that the disease can be controlled using methotrexate, hydroxychloroquine, allopurinol and cyclophosphamide but no large-scale research has been done on this subject.

WHAT TO EXPECT

About half the people who develop this disease will have a natural remission without any treatment, and there are generally no significant long-term complications. Although you might develop problems with your organs, this is usually minimal and not progressive. Recurrences of sarcoidosis occur in about 20 per cent of people with the disease.

CHAPTER | II

SJOGREN'S SYNDROME

I n 1933, a Swedish eye doctor, Henrik Sjogren, described a condition in which there is a slowly progressive inflammation of the lacrimal and salivary glands leading to dry eyes and a dry mouth. The inflammation is a result of stimulation of the immune system, which acts as if these glands are germs and tries to destroy them—usually very successfully.

Sjogren's syndrome can also affect other organs in the body and occasionally develops a cancer of the lymph glands (lymphoma). Sjogren's syndrome is classified as primary when it happens spontaneously, or secondary when it's associated with other inflammatory arthritic conditions, such as rheumatoid arthritis, lupus and scleroderma.

SJOGREN'S SYNDROME CAUSES DRY EYES AND A DRY MOUTH BECAUSE IT ATTACKS THE LACRIMAL AND SALIVARY GLANDS.

STATITISTICS AND CAUSES OF SJOGREN'S SYNDROME

Nine times more women get the disease at any age, but it's more common in middle age. Less than 1 per cent of the population will develop the primary form, but almost one-third of inflammatory arthritis sufferers will develop secondary Sjogren's syndrome.

The immune cells (B and T lymphocytes) infiltrate the tissues and release protein antibodies that stimulate the attack on the body's tissues causing inflammation. Two of these antibodies (Ro/SS-A and La/SS-B) can be used to help in the diagnosis. If they are present in the blood it usually indicates the disease will have an earlier age of onset, will last longer and be associated with vasculitis (inflammation of the blood vessels)and enlarged salivary glands.

Genetics

If you get Sjogren's syndrome you'll have a genetic susceptibility. The genetic markers associated with primary Sjogren's syndrome (HLA-B8, HLA-DR3 and HLA-DQA1 0501) are probably stimulated by a viral infection.

FEATURES OF SJOGREN'S SYNDROME

If you have primary Sjogren's syndrome, you'll have a slow, relatively quiet disease for 10 years before you experience full-blown symptoms, such as swollen salivary glands. Your organs may also be affected—this occurs in one-third of people with the disease.

The eyes

You'll notice that the cornea of the eye dries out and becomes scratchy, red and irritable. This is because the disease affects the lacrimal gland, which supplies tears for the eyes. Tears supply the cornea with nutrients. (The cornea doesn't have its own blood supply—if it did, the blood vessels would make the cornea opaque and you wouldn't be able to see.)

The body tries to compensate for the lack of nutrients by producing more tears, so you can also get a watery eye at the same time. But despite these tears, your eye is still nutrient deficent and your cornea gets more inflamed and may become ulcerated. An eye specialist can measure tear production using a Schirmer's test.

Salivary glands

The salivary glands are affected in the same way as the lacrimal glands, resulting in decreased saliva production and enlarged salivary glands. Saliva initiates digestion and breakdown of food when we chew. Saliva is also important in maintaining mouth hygiene as it digests and breaks down food particles caught between our teeth (like a chemical dental floss).

Saliva also contains the immune proteins immunoglobulin A, which is a first line protection against infections. Without saliva, the mouth is an unhealthy environment and is prone to infections, dental caries and nerve damage, all of which can lead to a chronic painful mouth with a loss of taste. When the salivary glands become inflamed in Sjogren's syndrome they tend to become swollen and painful. This occurs in about two-thirds of people with primary Sjogren's syndrome, but is uncommon in secondary Sjogren's syndrome.

THE SALIVARY GLANDS BECOME SWOLLEN AND PAINFUL AND SALIVA PRODUCTION DECREASES, MAKING YOUR MOUTH MORE SUSCEPTIBLE TO INFECTIONS.

Other organs
About 60 per cent of people with Sjogren's syndrome also have associated arthritis at some stage of the disease, but the arthritis is usually non-destructive. You're most likely to experience generalised symptoms such as fatigue and low grade fevers. Your lungs might also be affected but this is rarely bad enough to cause symptoms. The kidneys can become inflamed or accumulate calcium deposits. Vasculitis (inflammation of the blood vessels) can also damage the kidney as well as leading to skin ulcers, rashes, nerve damage, and in some cases induce strokes or convulsions.

Lymphomas occur in 5 per cent of people with primary Sjogren's syndrome and appear as gland enlargement anywhere within the body, even in the lungs and gut—these are different from the original salivary gland swelling. In mild Sjogren's disease you can develop lymphomas, but these are more likely if the disease is affecting organs other than the salivary and lacrimal glands.

TREATMENT OF SJOGREN'S SYNDROME
Although there is no cure for Sjogren's syndrome, you can help your symptoms by using lubricating nutrient drops and gels for the eyes, and

frequent artificial saliva and mouth washes and analgesics. Hydroxychloroquine may help with the arthritis and if your lungs or kidneys are affected you can use cortisone.

WHAT TO EXPECT

Generally the outlook for those with Sjogren's syndrome is good and the vast majority of those affected live normal lives without significant problems. Any that arise are usually mild, tend to remain stable and rarely progress. The mortality rate with the disease is only about 2 per cent.

SERO-NEGATIVE ARTHRITIS

S ero-negative arthritises are forms of arthritis that don't have a blood test marker to help in diagnosis. The most common types are psoriatic arthritis, ankylosing spondylitis, reactive arthritis and Reiter's syndrome. From my perspective it also lumps together those conditions that look like a particular disease but for which the blood tests for that condition are negative.

PSORIATIC ARTHRITIS

Psoriasis is a disease in which the skin becomes inflamed from an immune stimulation. The result is often extensive plaques of thickened, scaly skin that usually sheds dead, white, dandruff-like material. Although this is a skin disease, in some people it can develop a significant complication—chronic inflammatory arthritis. Like most inflammatory arthritis the cause is unknown but has a genetic basis with a possible infectious or drug-related triggering factor. Psoriasis-like conditions can be induced by both the drug interferon, and the human immunodeficiency virus (HIV).

Features of psoriatic arthritis

The symptoms of psoriatic arthritis vary, but it typically affects the finger joints causing the fingers to take on a sausage shape. The hips, knees and ankles are the next most common joints affected. You're likely to notice the skin rash for some years before any other symptoms. Your fingernails will look pitted and small divots develop in the nails themselves, distinguishing it from rheumatoid arthritis. If you have asymmetrical psoriatic arthritis (occurring in about half of cases), your outlook is good, as there is only a 25 per cent chance of developing joint destruction or eye inflammation.

THE FINGER JOINTS ARE TYPICALLY AFFECTED IN PSORIATIC ARTHRITIS. THE FINGERNAILS ALSO TAKE ON A PITTED APPEARANCE.

About one-quarter of psoriatic arthritis patients develop an arthritis similar in distribution to rheumatoid, symmetrically on the hand and wrist. Large joints such as hips, knees and shoulders can also be affected. Women are twice as likely as men to get the disease, which is destructive unless you get proper treatment.

One-quarter of people with psoriatic arthritis develop a spondylitis (arthritis of the lower back) and inflamed sacroiliac joints (the joints between the pelvis and the lower part of the spine, the sacrum). More men get this type of arthritis, which often results in lower back pain and morning back stiffness. You may have a psoriasis rash for several years before the back complaint develops. Other joints may or may not be affected and because it progresses slowly, the arthritis is generally not destructive. Tendons are particularly affected by inflammation in this form, especially the Achilles tendon at the back of the heel.

The pathology of psoriatic arthritis is similar to rheumatoid, with the cells of the synovium being involved in the inflammation process. This is especially so if the psoriatic arthritis has a destructive tendency. You may also develop fibrosis or scarring of the joint capsule and bone marrow.

There are no specific blood tests for psoriatic arthritis but your doctor will usually be able to make a clear-cut diagnosis, although it can be difficult to diagnose if you don't have these symptoms, especially if there is no nail pitting or psoriasis rash. I once missed the diagnosis when my patient complained of a sore knee. He had no psoriasis rash except for a small 1 cm patch between his buttocks. It's not often that a doctor examines someone's buttocks to reach a diagnosis of arthritis! Psoriatic rashes may be small and can also be hidden in the scalp and belly button. If your doctor doesn't find a psoriasis rash, he or she will diagnose by excluding other forms of arthritis.

X-rays of the hands do show some unique features. Bone erosions at the finger joints closest to the finger tips, bony expansion of the base of the bone of the finger tip (the distal phalanx) and bony overgrowth or tufting of the end of the distal phalanx confirms the diagnosis.

Treatment of psoriatic arthritis

To relieve your symptoms you can take non-steroidal anti-inflammatories and analgesics. If the arthritis is destructive to a joint, long-term disease-modifying drugs are the best option. Methotrexate is usually the drug first chosen because as well as helping the arthritis, methotrexate also helps the skin rash. Other disease-modifying drugs used include sulfasalazine, gold, cyclosporin, azathioprine and hydroxychloroquine, although hydroxychloroquine may aggravate the rash.

ANKYLOSING SPONDYLITIS

Ankylosing spondylitis is an inflammatory arthritis that usually affects the spine and larger joints of the body and sometimes other body organs. Men are three times more likely than women to get the disease, which often starts in the 20 to 30 year-old age group. A small number of people get spondylitis in adolescence—the hips are usually severely affected and the outlook is worse than in the adult-onset disease. In general, ankylosing spondylitis ranges from mild stiffness to a total spine fusion from the buttocks to the base of the skull associated with eye and heart problems. If you get ankylosing spondylitis you'll most likely live a normal life with only a minimal risk of life-threatening complications affecting either the kidney, heart or lungs.

Ankylosing spondylitis has a strong genetic basis and in 90 per cent of people is associated with the genetic marker, HLA B-27. This marker occurs in only 7 per cent of the general population. HLA B-27 is not a disease marker as it doesn't fluctuate with disease activity. It's not specific to ankylosing spondylitis as it occurs in many other diseases.

Like other inflammatory arthritis there must also be a triggering factor for the disease. It's thought that some bacteria from within the bowel, such as *klebsiella pneumoniae,* may trigger ankylosing spondylitis. It's also associated with inflammatory bowel diseases such as Crohn's disease and ulcerative colitis (see Chapter 15).

X-ray changes of the spine can help in diagnosis, but as spinal changes occur later in the disease, early diagnosis by X-ray is difficult.

Features of ankylosing spondylitis

The sacroiliac joint between the lower spine and the pelvis is usually the first joint to become inflamed. The result is cartilage destruction and bone hardening (sclerosis). Eventually the sacroiliac joint is destroyed and the joint fuses. As the disease progresses the disc cartilage between the vertebrae and the margins of the vertebral bone become inflamed and the outer fibres of the disc are replaced by bone. A bony bridge (syndesmophytes) forms between the vertebrae. (This shows up clearly on an X-ray of the spine.) Syndesmophytes form up the spine from bottom to top and if several vertebrae are affected, the X-ray shows a series of episodic flowing protrusions along the length of spine, like a length of bamboo.

The inflammation of ankylosing spondylitis then goes on to involve the spine's facet joints that help with the body's rotational movements. The vertebral bone loses calcium and the bone becomes osteoporotic and soft. Joints affected by ankylosing spondylitis have synovial inflammation and overgrowth with pannus formation, but this is much less severe than it is in rheumatoid arthritis. Tendon insertions on bone can also be inflamed in ankylosing spondylitis. A very small percentage of patients with this disease can develop scar tissue within the heart resulting in valve problems and abnormal heart beats.

THE SPINE IS OFTEN AFFECTED BY ANKYLOSING SPONDYLITIS.

You'll usually get symptoms in early adulthood. Lower back pain with stiffness in the spine lasting up to several hours is often the first symptom. The pain improves when you move and it may be worse at night. About one third of people with spondylitis have arthritis of the hips and shoulders. Later it may affect your spine and later your neck. Because ankylosing spondylitis is inflammatory, you may experience generalised symptoms of fevers, weight loss, loss of appetite, fatigue and sweats. Although about 50 per cent of people may have a bowel inflammation, it usually isn't bad enough to bring on symptoms. Fibrosis and scarring of the lungs are rare.

When ankylosing spondylitis affects the spine, the main thing you'll notice is a loss of mobility of the spine and associated stiffness. You won't be able to bend and touch your toes or turn your spine and look sideways. The spine loses its intrinsic curves as the vertebrae fuse and the muscles often go into spasm, further decreasing spinal mobility. As the disease progresses, your posture becomes a characteristic feature of the disease—a stooping forward of the head and neck, an exaggeration of the forward curve of the spine of the chest and a loss of the curve of the lower part of the spine.

Because ankylosing spondylitis is associated with osteoporosis of the spine, there is risk of vertebral fractures from minor trauma with the associated risk of spinal cord paralysis. The neck is most commonly involved, and quadriplegia the worst possible outcome.

Treatment of ankylosing spondylitis

Unfortunately, treatment options are limited. Mobilisation exercises are most important from an early stage of the disease to maintain spine flexibility. Drug treatment options are somewhat limited. Non-steroidal anti-inflammatory medications appear to settle inflammation and symptoms. Sulfasalazine has been proven to modify the disease activity and methotrexate may also help, but other disease-modifying agents don't work. The long-term use of cortisone is not recommended because of the risk of osteoporosis, although X-ray guided injections into the sacroiliac and spinal joints often settle symptoms for some time. Surgery is usually limited to hip replacements or stabilisation of the neck spine at the base of the skull if necessary. Eye complications such as anterior uveitis (inflammation of the front chamber of the eye) respond to cortisone drops in the eyes.

REACTIVE ARTHRITIS AND REITER'S SYNDROME

As its name suggests, reactive arthritis happens as a reaction to something else, usually an infection. The infection doesn't directly involve the joint and yet the joint suffers an acute flare-up of arthritis. You might, for example, have an infection in the bowel or the urinary tract with the side effect of a concurrent joint inflammation. Although the joint isn't infected (it doesn't contain any microorganisms), the inflammation happens because of the generalised immune reaction induced by the bug, which then also affects the joint.

In reactive arthritis, white blood cells (lymphocytes) which specifically respond to proteins of the invading infective microorganism, are found in the synovium in the joints. Probably the most well known example is rheumatic fever, in which a throat infected with *streptococcus* induces inflammation (but not infection) of joints, kidneys and heart valves.

REACTIVE ARTHRITIS IS AN ACUTE FLARE-UP OF ARTHRITIS CAUSED BY AN INFECTION SOMEWHERE ELSE IN THE BODY

Reactive arthritis is usually genetically determined with a strong correlation with HLA B-27, the same genetic marker associated with ankylosing spondylitis. Aproximately 75 per cent of people with reactive arthritis test positive for this marker. Like so many other forms of arthritis, the cause is exposure to an environmental factor, in this case an infection, in a genetically susceptible person. The two most common are bowel (with *shigella, salmonella, yersinia* and *campylobacter* species) and urinary tract infections (with *chlamydia trachomatis*).

Reactive arthritis is common in the 20 to 40 year age group but can also affect children and the elderly. Reactive arthritis secondary to bowel infections equally affects men and women (about 3.5 cases per 100,000 population). This figure may increase to one case per 1,000 in sub-populations that are especially affected by bowel and venereal infections, such as urban homosexual males. HIV in HLA B-27 positive people will especially result in a very aggressive form of reactive arthritis.

There is no specific blood test or X-ray findings that confirm the diagnosis of reactive arthritis and your doctor will base the diagnosis on the history of infections and following symptoms. Blood test or faecal serology may be helpful in pinpointing what infection precipitated the arthritis, but treating that infection doesn't usually help the arthritis. This is because the arthritis is non-infectious and is caused by flaws in the functioning of the immune system. It's important to exclude infective arthritis secondary to the gonorrhoea bacteria from NSU-induced reactive arthritis, as both give inflammation of the urethra but gonorrhoea infective arthritis needs to be treated with antibiotics.

Reiter's syndrome

Reiter's syndrome is a form of reactive arthritis with associated inflammation of the urethra (the exit tube from the bladder) and the conjunctiva in the eye. It's usually caused by *chlamydia trachomatis,* which is considered to be a male-oriented venereal disease also known as non-specific urethritis or NSU. It tends to last a lot longer than other types of reactive arthritis.

Features of reactive arthritis

With reactive arthritis you may have a short-term arthritis affecting only one joint ranging to a severe arthritis affecting many joints and organs. You may have also have had an infection one to four weeks before the arthritis began. Symptoms include loss of energy, fever and weight loss. The arthritis usually occurs suddenly, and is cumulative, with a new joint being involved every week or so. Reactive arthritis seems to prefer the joints of the legs and feet—tendons and other soft tissues of the joint also become inflamed.

Your eyes can be affected—from a benign conjunctivitis to uveitis (an inflammation of the front part of the eye) potentially resulting in loss of sight—you'll need cortisone to calm this down. You may also get mouth ulcers and thickened blisters on the palms of the hand and the soles of the feet and rarely heart and lung complications.

How long the arthritis lasts and the future recurrence rate of the reactive arthritis depends on the type of micro-organism infecting you. *Yersinia* bowel infection has a lower rate of chronic flare-ups than other infections, but generally somewhere between 30 to 60 per cent of people with reactive arthritis experience chronic recurrences of their arthritis, and about one-quarter of these suffer a severe disability.

Treatment of reactive arthritis

To treat reactive arthritis you'll need to take non-steroidal anti-inflammatory medications and analgesics for the pain, and sulfasalazine for disease suppression. Azathioprine and methotrexate may help if you have severe unresponsive disease, and you may need cortisone to settle severe symptoms quickly. The question of treating the actual infective micro-organism is debatable because by the time the arthritis has developed, the disease has usually been eliminated from the body. If the micro-organism can be identified in the infective stage, then there is some evidence to suggest that killing the micro-organism quicker, by giving antibiotics, decreases the chance of reactive arthritis developing.

WHAT TO EXPECT

Psoriatic arthritis is usually not life threatening as it tends not to affect major organs such as the heart, lungs or kidneys. Only one-quarter of people who have the condition suffer permanent destruction of their joints. The outlook for ankylosing spondylitis is less positive. Most people with this disease lead normal, full lives, but a small number have a reduced life expectancy due to fractures of the spine, with damage to the spinal cord, or heart or kidney complications. The outlook for people suffering from a reactive arthritis varies, depending on the type of infection and the organs affected. Reactive arthritis from HIV has a poor prognosis, not so much because of the arthritis but because of the serious infection. The same applies to rheumatic fever in which the heart and kidneys are affected. Up to one-half of those with reactive arthritis may have persisting arthritis symptoms five or more years later.

CHAPTER | 13

GOUTY ARTHRITIS

M ost people chuckle when someone they know has an attack of gout, but in spite of popular belief, gout is not necessarily related to drinking alcohol, or eating tomatoes or spicy food.

Gout is a metabolic disease in which there is either an overproduction in the body of the substance urate or uric acid, or in which there is a decreased clearance of urate from the body. Both conditions lead to too much urate, which crystallises out of the blood and serum and deposits itself in a joint, causing gouty arthritis. The process of crystallisation is similar to putting too much sugar in your tea. Some of the sugar dissolves but some remains as a crystal at the bottom of the cup, as the tea is saturated with sugar. Too much urate in a joint leads to excruciating pain. Between 2 to 13 per cent of adults have high blood levels of urate and the incidence of gouty arthritis is between 1.5 per cent to 4 per cent.

Urate is the end product of purine breakdown in the body. Purine is an essential chemical used in the building blocks of genes and also in the chemicals that produce energy for the cells. It's continually being broken down and reused. Purine is used in all tissues but urate is only produced in the liver and small intestine. The level of urate in the blood depends on:

▶ the amount of purine you ingest in food
▶ the amount of purine broken down in cells
▶ the amount of urate removed by the kidneys.

Normally, the kidneys remove 70 per cent of urate and the rest is removed by the small intestines. Any conditions influencing urate production or removal from the body also influence the development of gouty arthritis.

URIC ACID IS ONE OF THE BODY'S WASTE PRODUCTS. WHEN THERE IS EXCESS URIC ACID IN THE BODY, IT CAN RESULT IN AN INFLAMMATION OF THE JOINTS. THIS IS GOUT.

High levels of urate in the blood, hyperuricaemia, can lead to gouty arthritis, tophaceous gout (in which urate is deposited in and around joint tissues), kidney disease and kidney stones. Crystals are not necessarily formed when there are high levels of urate in the blood. You could have hyperuricaemia and no symptoms at all—you will only get symptoms if there is crystal formation. Levels of urate in the blood rise steadily as you get older and can vary with height, body weight, diet, blood pressure, kidney function and liver function. This is why gout tends to happen as you get older—men are also more likely than women to get gout. Women are protected to a degree by female hormones; once they reach menopause, the urate levels do a rapid catch-up to male levels. If your body fluid is acidic, it's also likely that crystals will form. Acidic urine is a factor in the development of kidney disease and kidney stones.

Urate may be more likely to crystallise in a joint with damaged cartilage due to the release of mucopolysaccharides and other chemicals into the joint fluid.

FEATURES OF GOUTY ARTHRITIS
Gout in a joint has a very rapid onset and is exceedingly painful. It may be preceded by a dull ache in the joint for a few hours before it flares up, and usually it only affects one joint at a time, although women can be affected

in several joints at once. The pain of gout is coupled with a very red, swollen, hot joint that is exquisitely tender to touch. If left untreated, the attack peaks at one to two days and subsides in about 10 days.

Gouty arthritis prefers to attack joints of the legs and feet, and as well as affecting the actual joints can also inflame tendon insertion points on bones such as the Achilles tendon, the bursae of joints, especially at the elbow, and the soft tissue of the arch of the foot. The joint between the big toe and the foot is often the first joint affected, especially if you already have a bunion there. The second most common site for a gout attack is the hand and finger joints, followed by the wrists and elbows.

Any abrupt change of urate levels in the blood, either up or down, is thought to induce gout. A sudden increase in urate is also thought to produce new crystals of urate leading to a flare-up of gout and a sudden decrease of urate levels to shedding of previously formed crystals within a joint, resulting in a flare-up. The sudden decrease in urate levels explains why when you have been treated for a long time, you can get a flare up before the gout settles again.

CAUSES OF GOUTY ARTHRITIS

Urate overproduction, decreased urate clearance from the body, or a combination of both are the causes of gout.

Increased urate production

The main cause of high urate production is the high intake of purine in the diet. Purine is present to a higher degree in red and white meat, liver, kidney and anchovy so if you suffer from gout, avoid these foods. Medically, gout is the only type of arthritis in which diet has been proven to make any difference to the outcome of the disease.

GOUT IS THE ONLY TYPE OF ARTHRITIS IN WHICH DIET HAS BEEN PROVEN TO MAKE A DIFFERENCE.

Genetic diseases can also lead to over production of urate. Often associated with brain disorders, they are not common and usually involve enzyme deficiencies or enzyme overactivity within cells. Conditions that lead to rapid cell turnover in the body also lead to excess urate production.

Purine is released from your cells and urate is then produced in excess quantities. Some examples of rapid cell turnover-inducing gout are leukemia, chemotherapy for cancers, psoriasis, haemolytic anaemia and widespread muscle breakdown from marathon-type sports.

Decreased urate clearance

The kidney is responsible for getting rid of urate from the body—almost everyone who develops gout has a defect in the kidney's ability to remove urate. It is this defect—and not alcohol—that predominantly gives people gout. If you have gout, your kidneys are around 40 per cent less efficient than in normal people. Kidney efficiency is also lowered if there is an underlying kidney disease of another cause. Even gout itself can damage the kidney, which then increases the gout tendency.

ALMOST EVERYONE WHO HAS GOUT HAS A DEFECT IN THEIR KIDNEYS' ABILITY TO REMOVE URATE.

Alcohol can influence the onset of a gout attack by bringing on the production of chemicals, which are then cleared from the body by the kidney at the same sites from which urate is cleared. If these sites are being used by alcohol by-products, there are no spaces left for urate clearance in the kidney, and the urate stays inside you. This leads to gout. The same process can happen in uncontrolled diabetes, starvation and aspirin overdose.

Combined mechanisms

Alcohol is the most common cause of both increased urate production and decreased urate clearance from the body. If you drink too much alcohol, purine and urate production will increase in the liver and at the same time lactic acid levels in the blood increase, blocking clearance of the urate by the kidney. Some alcohol, such as beer, also has a high purine content. Some hereditary conditions involving enzyme deficiencies also increase urate production and decrease urate clearance—this can bring on gout at an early age.

Other factors involved in gouty arthritis

Stress, trauma, infection, surgery, starvation and weight reduction, excessive food intake, alcohol and some medications, especially diuretics (drugs designed to remove fluid from the body used especially in the treatment of high blood pressure and heart failure) can also bring on an attack of gouty arthritis.

OTHER COMPLICATIONS OF HIGH URATE

If you have high levels of urate in the body, you won't usually have any symptoms until you get gouty arthritis; deposits of urate 'tophi' in the kidney (tophaceous gout); and possibly kidney stones. The higher the level of urate in the blood the higher your risk of getting gouty arthritis. The complications of gout relate to both how long the urate has been in your body and how severe it is—most people have their first episode of gouty arthritis 20 to 40 years after high levels of urate first develop. Most men get gout at 40 to 60 and women after menopause.

Acute gout

Acute gout is the result of an interaction between urate crystals and white blood cells (neutrophils). The neutrophils are stimulated by the urate crystals to release enzymes and other inflammatory proteins that give the severe inflammation of gouty arthritis, which leads to cartilage and bone damage. Some of the released proteins then increase the urate effect on the neutrophils, making the whole episode twice as bad. The tophi of chronic gouty arthritis are chalky collections of urate crystals with a surrounding inflammatory reaction initiated by other white blood cells (phagocytes), the scavenger cells of the immune system. Tophi can also destroy cartilage, bone and surrounding joint tissue.

Urate-induced kidney disease

The most common kidney problem caused by high urate levels in the blood is kidney stones (in which urate accumulates in small patches) which start from a gravel and develop into a stone. When kidney stones break away from the kidney and try to pass down the ureter (the narrow tube joining the kidney and bladder), the muscle of the ureter cramps, causing severe pain. The kidney stone can also obstruct the ureter and may need surgical removal. Kidney stones can also be the focus of repeated bacterial infection, and you may need to take frequent doses of antibiotics until the stone is removed. If you suffer from gouty arthritis and kidney stones, the kidney stones often come before the arthritis.

Urate nephropathy, the other kidney problem associated with high urate levels, leads to kidney failure. A late feature of severe gout, it happens when urate crystals deposit in the kidney tissue and become inflamed. The kidney tissue has a very fine filter structure and the urate crystals physically block the kidney's microscopic tubes and filters. The urate also causes an inflammatory reaction within the kidney tissue and this destroys the filter system, eventually resulting in kidney failure. Having inflamed urate areas of the kidney also increases the chance of severe kidney infections. This complication of gout is now rare, because current treatments decrease the amount of urate in the body. Before these treatments became available, kidney failure was the cause of death in 25 per cent of people with gout.

Rapid urate production, resulting in blockage of the microscopic filtration tubes of the kidney tissue, can also bring on kidney failure. This is common in leukemia—a symptom of leukemia may actually be a flare up of gouty arthritis. Other causes are dehydration, severe prolonged epileptic seizures, vigorous exercise and severe diabetes. With the right treatment the survival rate is doubled.

INVESTIGATIONS INTO GOUTY ARTHRITIS

You will only need two investigations for the diagnosis of gout. First, your doctor will determine the blood level of urate, as the diagnosis of gout is rarely appropriate if your initial blood urate level is normal. Next your doctor will analyse joint fluid for urate crystals, providing he or she is able to get fluid from the inflamed joint. The fluid is examined through a microscope under polarised light—if the cause is gout, gout crystals will be present.

TO CONFIRM A DIAGNOSIS OF GOUT, YOUR DOCTOR WILL TEST FOR URATE LEVELS IN THE BLOOD, AND ANALYSE JOINT FLUID FOR URATE CRYSTALS.

TREATMENT FOR GOUTY ARTHRITIS

The treatment regime chosen for gout depends on how severe your gout is and how often it recurs. There are treatments for acute flare-up as well as those to protect against further flare-ups. If you're only having one attack every six months it's probably not worth taking tablets every day. If the attacks are more frequent, the likelihood of having complications of gout and the disruption to your life warrants using daily medications to ward off gout attacks.

Drugs used for gout

Some drugs that are only used for gout and aren't usually of any use in other types of arthritis include colchicine, allopurinol, probenecid and sulfinpyrazone.

Colchicine

An older drug that acts as an anti-inflammatory, colchicine gives a rapid relief of the inflammation of gout. It has no effect on the blood levels of urate, or its clearance from the body by the kidneys, and its long-term use doesn't prevent gout-induced kidney disease. Colchicine works in gout inflammation by inhibiting the action of immune-related white blood cells (neutrophils), the cells stimulated by urate crystals to give inflammation.

Colchicine is highly effective in settling gout symptoms but isn't tolerated well in higher doses. The initial recommended dose is 1000 mcg orally, followed by 500 mcg every two hours until the pain has settled. With this dose about 90 per cent of people experience abdominal pain, nausea and diarrhoea—a smaller initial dose followed by 500 mcg two or three times a day settles the gout over a day or so. The larger dose works more quickly but is not helpful if you can't tolerate the side effects, particularly if you're elderly or frail, but if you're otherwise healthy, you should be able to tolerate the lower doses. Unlike non-steroidal anti-inflammatory medications, colchinine won't bring on stomach ulcers.

You can also use colchicine for chronic, recurring gout as a preventive for acute flare-ups. The typical dose is 500 mcg twice daily—you may be able to tolerate this better than non-steroidals.

Allopurinol

Allopurinol has become a lifesaver for people with chronic gout—because of this drug people with gout no longer suffer kidney disease and premature death. Joint destruction is also lessened as allopurinol decreases the blood urate levels very effectively.

Allopurinol decreases urate levels in the blood by interfering with an enzyme in the liver and small intestine cells (*xanthine oxidase*), which helps break down purine. The result is that less urate is formed in the body and there is a lower level of urate in the blood and joint fluid. The likelihood of urate over-saturation and crystal formation is markedly decreased. The crystals and tophi that have already formed are slowly re-dissolved back into the body's fluids and removed from the body.

The major drawback is that if you take it when your gouty arthritis is active or even if there's a minor gout-induced inflammation, the gout will flare up—the rapid decrease in blood levels of urate will lead to crystal shedding within the joint. You can overcome this problem by having a total gout-free period of six weeks before you start allopurinol. Do this by using allopurinol in combination with colchinine or a non-steroidal for three months as a protection against a flare-up. Once the three months is up, use allopurinol by itself and you're unlikely to get further gouty arthritis attacks.

Generally speaking, allopurinol is well tolerated once you overcome the possible initial flare-up of gouty arthritis. Although rare, known side effects include skin rashes and other allergic reactions. If you experience these, don't use allopurinol again.

There have been occasional reports of liver damage, kidney inflammation, nausea and vomiting (when allopurinol is taken on an empty stomach), malaise, changed bowel habit, headache, vertigo, lack of muscle/nerve coordination, impotence, loss of hair, slowing of the heart rate and high blood pressure. All these side effects are very uncommon but you should use allopurinol in conjunction with azathioprine with caution, because of the interactions between the two drugs. Allopurinol may also interact with cyclosporin—you will need to adjust the dose. If you use the antibiotic amoxycillin at the same time you may get a skin rash.

THE SIDE EFFECTS OF ALLOPURINOL,
WHILE POTENTIALLY SEVERE, ARE RARE.

The usual dose for healthy adults is 300 mg daily orally. Some very severe cases may need up to 900 mg daily. If you are elderly or frail, your kidney clearance rates are slower and you may need a smaller dose of 100 mg daily.

Probenecid
Probenecid doesn't lower urate production in the body, but it does increase the clearance of urate by stopping the kidney reabsorbing the urate once

in the urine. By increasing clearance of urate from the body, urate levels are lowered and eventually the crystals and tophi are reabsorbed. Most people with chronic, recurring, gouty arthritis find it effective, especially if there's a hereditary defect in urate clearance from the kidney. Probenecid may also improve kidney function by helping to remove any urate deposits from the kidney itself.

As with allopurinol, don't start using probenecid during an acute flare-up of gouty arthritis. You can use it in combination with allopurinol. You must not use it in combination with methotrexate as it can increase the blood levels of this drug, and is potentially dangerous. It also increases the blood levels of penicillin antibiotics, sometimes used medically to treat resistant infections.

Possible side effects of probenecid use include headache, nausea, loss of appetite, increased urination, skin rashes, hair loss, allergic reactions, dizziness, anaemia and kidney problems. These side effects are uncommon and most people tolerate the drug well. The usual dose of probenecid is up to 500 mg twice daily orally. Unfortunately, this drug has been removed from the market in Australia as the drug company found it uneconomical to distribute.

Sulfinpyrazone
Similar in its effect to probenecid, sulfinpyrazone increases the amount of urate thrown out of the body into the urine by stopping the reabsorption of urate from the urine by the kidney. Like the other urate blood level lowering drugs, don't take it if your gouty arthritis is playing up.

SOME OF THE DRUGS USED FOR GOUT SHOULDN'T BE TAKEN WHEN THE ARTHRITIS IS FLARING UP.

Sulfinpyrazone is usually only used by people with persistent gouty problems—allopurinol and probenecid are much safer drugs. Its side effects include bleeding gastric ulcers, nausea, vomiting, diarrhoea, kidney failure, allergic reactions, bone marrow suppression and liver problems. If you have a history of stomach ulcers, liver, kidney or bone marrow problems you shouldn't take it. Your doctor should also regularly monitor these organs through blood tests.

Sulfinpyrazone has also been known to interact with blood-thinning drugs, diabetes medications, other sulphur drugs, penicillins and aspirin, so use it carefully if you're taking other drugs. The usual dose is 200 to 400 mg daily in three to four divided doses orally. You can take it in combination with allopurinol.

Treatment for acute attacks

If you have an acute flare-up of gout your doctor will recommend similar treatments to those for acute flare-ups of other types of arthritis. Because the pain of gout is severe, you'll often need stronger narcotic pain killers. Rest is very important, as is minimal use of the inflamed joint. Non-steroidal anti-inflammatory medications are usually effective in settling the redness, swelling and pain within a few days. If you can't tolerate non-steroidals or have had peptic ulcers you can take cox-2 inhibitors and colchinine. Joint injections with cortisone-type drugs will also quickly relieve your symptoms. Some specialist rheumatologists recommend low-dose cortisone to cut down the inflammation.

Treatment for recurring gout

The basis of treatment for recurring gout is to keep the blood urate levels low. There are several drugs that can be used to do this, one of the most common being allopurinol. Allopurinol inhibits the production of urate within the cells while the other drugs (probenecid and sulfinpyrazone) lower blood urate levels by increasing clearance of urate through the kidney into the urine. Excess urate production is a lifelong problem, so the use of urate-lowering drugs is also lifelong. If your condition isn't controlled on allopurinol alone, you can use a combination of urate-lowering drugs. By keeping the urate level as low as possible you substantially reduce the risk of recurring gout and kidney problems from urate and prevent death caused by kidney failure.

THE RISK OF RECURRING GOUT AND KIDNEY PROBLEMS IS MINIMISED BY KEEPING THE URATE LEVEL AS LOW AS POSSIBLE.

A low protein diet, which is low in purine, will help you control your gout and its consequences. If you find that alcohol aggravates your gout avoid it, or at least drink less. Beer is high in purine content so it is best to avoid it entirely.

*AVOID BEER IF YOU SUFFER FROM GOUT,
AS IT HAS A HIGH PURINE CONTENT.*

PSEUDOGOUT AND CRYSTAL ARTHRITIS

Before the advent of crystal analysis techniques in rheumatology, many gout-like attacks were diagnosed as gout, when in fact other types of crystals caused the arthritis. These other crystals are calcium pyrophosphate dihydrate (CPPD), calcium hydroxyapatite (HA) and calcium oxalate (CaOx). CPPD is the most common and was the original crystal used for the term pseudogout (which looks and feels like gout but isn't). It deposits itself in cartilage, synovium, ligaments and tendons and frequently affects the elderly (up to 15 per cent of the 65 to 75 age group and up to 60 per cent of the over 85s).

It's thought the pre-existing joint damage from other conditions, such as osteoarthritis, and chemical changes in ageing cartilage bring on the formation of CPPD crystals. Like urate crystals in a joint, these crystals stimulate the immune system's white blood cells (neutrophils) resulting in inflammation of the joint.

CPPD-induced pseudogout can also result from the production of CPPD crystals in some types of uncommon diseases, such as hyperparathyroidism (excess parathyroid hormone), haemochromatosis (iron overload) and hypophosphataemia (low phosphate levels in the blood). These diseases may cause pseudogout in younger people.

*PSEUDOGOUT IS MORE COMMON IN OLDER ADULTS,
USUALLY OVER THE AGE OF 65.*

You may not have any symptoms with CPPD pseudogout, but it has many similarities to gout in its distribution and symptoms (if you have them). However, if left untreated, it doesn't lead to kidney failure or kidney stones. The complications of CPPD pseudogout include the development of secondary osteoarthritis, synovitis that looks similar to rheumatoid arthritis synovitis, intervertebral disc and ligament calcification that mimics ankylosing spondylitis and, rarely, the compression of the spinal cord by the inflammation of the CPPD-induced arthritis. Most people will have at least five joints affected at some stage. To diagnose, your doctor will look for X-ray changes of the joint where calcification of the cartilage appears. Diagnosis is only confirmed by the examination of joint fluid where CPPD crystals are present.

A minor trauma, such as a sprain of a joint, can set off an attack of CPPD pseudogout. Fever might also cause the flare up, making the diagnosis difficult, as infective arthritis (see Chapter 14) needs to be excluded.

Treatment of CPPD pseudogout

Treatment of CPPD pseudogout is with non-steroidals, analgesics, joint injections with cortisone, and possibly colchicine. Unlike gout, there is no method of decreasing CPPD crystals within a joint by using an equivalent drug to allopurinol.

Other types of crystal arthritis

Hydroxyapatite (HA) is the primary mineral of bone and teeth. Abnormal collections can occur in areas of damaged tissue and can also be induced by hyperparathyroidism, ageing, osteoarthritis, long-term dialysis for kidney failure and scleroderma. The incidence of HA arthritis isn't known but up to half of people with osteoarthritis have HA crystals within the joint and HA arthritis may actually be the cause of so-called acute flare-ups of osteoarthritis. The most common sites of HA involvement are the knees, shoulders and finger joints. The arthritis can be most destructive and you may need joint replacement. Flare-ups of HA arthritis are treated the same way as CPPD pseudogout. There is also no allopurinol equivalent for long-term suppression of this disease. HA arthritis is not associated with kidney problems.

Calcium oxalate (CaOx) arthritis is the rarest type of crystal arthritis and is most often associated with severe kidney failure. You're more likely to get it if you have a kidney disease and are also taking vitamin C. This is because vitamin C is metabolised into oxalate and increases the chance of developing this disease. Calcium oxalate crystal is deposited in bone, cartilage, synovium and ligaments and can lead to joint destruction by overgrowth of synovium, which will destroy bone and cartilage. CaOx arthritis may be indistinguishable from other crystal arthropathies and can involve any joints within the body. Treatment of this disease is the same as for other forms of crystal arthritis and may also require maximisation of kidney function with dialysis.

WHAT TO EXPECT

Some people only have one attack of gout in their lifetime—the interval between first and second attacks is about two years for most people. If you have severe gouty arthritis you'll need long-term treatment or you could develop chronic tophaceous gout where deposits of urate (tophi) are formed in the soft tissues around a joint, in the cartilage of the ears and in the finger and toe pads as well as tendons. This takes approximately 10 years to develop after the first attack. If you have arthritis of tophaceous gout, your attacks will occur more frequently, last longer and will affect an increasing number of joints. Your arthritis can then become constant, although less severe, affecting many joints. If you have extremely high levels of urate in the blood, the bone and cartilage in your joints can be destroyed.

CHAPTER 14

INFECTIONS AND ARTHRITIS

Bacterial arthritis

Spirochetal arthritis

Mycobacterial arthritis

Fungal arthritis

Viral arthritis

Parasitic arthritis

S kin bugs, bowel bugs, tuberculosis, viruses, gonorrhoea, syphilis, various types of fungus, parasites, meningitis brain bugs and even a venereal disease of cows (brucellosis) can all cause arthritis.

But of all the micro-organisms to infect joints, the most common are the skin bacteria *Staphylococcus aureus* (golden staph) and *streptococcus* and the venereal disease *Neisseria gonorrhoeae*. Bacterial arthritis can quickly destroy the cartilage of a joint and, if you have any rapid onset of arthritis, your doctor needs to exclude the possibility of infection quickly to give you the best treatment and outlook. The exclusion of a joint infection can only be done by taking fluid from a joint and having the laboratory stain and culture it for micro-organisms. Usually infective arthritis from bacteria attacks only one or two joints at a time. Chronic arthritis that grumbles along may have been caused by tuberculosis infection or a fungus.

If you suffer from an underlying inflammatory arthritis, such as rheumatoid arthritis, you'll be predisposed to an infective arthritis. This is because the joint is chronically inflamed, and while cortisone treatments suppress the local immune reaction, there is often breakdown of skin from blood vessel inflammation, all of which mean you're more susceptible to infections. Diabetes, kidney dialysis, alcoholism, cancers, immune deficiencies and intravenous drug use also put you at greater risk of joint infection.

BACTERIAL ARTHRITIS

Bacteria usually enter a joint through the blood supply, although a penetrating wound into a joint can also do it. Any kind of wound to a joint needs to be meticulously cleaned and treated with antibiotics. When bacteria enter a joint they induce an immune reaction by white blood cells (neutrophils) within hours. It's often difficult to tell whether the joint is infected, or inflamed by gout, and as the results from the laboratory analysis of joint fluid may take some time, you may initially need treatment for both conditions.

A BACTERIAL INFECTION IN THE JOINT CAN DESTROY CARTILAGE WITHIN TWO DAYS, SO EARLY TREATMENT IS CRITICAL.

Destruction of the cartilage occurs within the first two days of infection and to minimise joint damage, it's essential you get early diagnosis and treatment. If you do have cartilage damage, you're at high risk of getting secondary osteoarthritis in 5 to 10 years' time. Microscopic studies of infected joints show that the bacteria adhere to the cartilage and synovium with, in severe cases, abscesses extending through the cartilage into the bone. The synovium is stimulated and overgrows the cartilage, further damaging it.

Different age, different bacteria

If the joints of children are infected, the most usual culprits are *group B* and *group A streptococci, Staphylococcus aureus* and some bacteria from the bowel such as *E. coli* and *klebsiella* species. In the adolescent and young adult age group the most common bacteria for joint infections is the gonorrhoea bacteria, and in adults, *Staphylococcus aureus*.

Of all the joints to be infected with bacteria, the knee is the most common site, and the great majority of people with bacterial arthritis are infected in only one joint. You'll usually feel severe pain, swelling of the joint and have a decreased range of movement and associated muscle spasm. Fever with temperatures higher than 38°C are common. X-rays initially only show soft tissue swelling and if there are changes of a narrowed joint space and bony erosions, the infection has been present for about six weeks and you'll certainly experience permanent and severe joint destruction.

Treatment of bacterial arthritis

You will need prompt surgery and intravenous antibiotics to clear the joint of infected material. The surgery is usually via arthroscopy and it's unusual to need to fully open the joint to clean it out, unless the infection is severe or the arthroscope cannot reach the joint (for example with the hips, joints of the spine, hands and toes). Until the complete laboratory analysis of joint fluid is done, your doctor will make an educated guess and prescribe you broad spectrum antibiotics to cover most possibilities. Once the bacteria (and its antibiotic sensitivity) are known, you will be prescribed the specific antibiotic.

Infective arthritis caused by *Neisseria gonorrhoeae* accounts for 70 per cent of cases in adults under the age of 40. It travels through the blood from the genital tract and mouth to the afflicted joint. Women are three times more likely to experience this than men. As well as inducing a direct infection of the joint, *Neisseria gonorrhoeae* can also give you an immune reaction leading to multiple joint arthritis, tenosynovitis and a rash. You will often have these symptoms before the joint is infected.

SPIROCHETAL ARTHRITIS

Spirochaetes are pygmy bacteria that can't be seen under normal microscopes and need immunofluorescent equipment or electron microscopes to be seen. The two that are relevant to arthritis are *Borrelia burgdorferi,* which leads to Lyme disease, and *Treponema pallidum,* which results in syphilis.

Lyme disease

Lyme disease is virtually impossible to diagnose in its infective state because the initial symptoms are so non-specific. But if it isn't treated with antibiotics at this point, about 70 per cent of people with it will go on to develop arthritic complaints. The spirochaete is transferred to the human by a tick bite (from the *Ixodes* variety). Although Lyme disease is more common in North America, it's also found along the east coast of Australia.

The large joints can become infected, especially the knee. Many people have symptoms that come and go over a number of months, and about 15 per cent of people per year find the arthritis resolves itself, but about 10 per cent develop chronic arthritis with erosion and destruction of the joint.

Syphilis

Syphilis can bring on arthritis at different stages of its disease course. If syphilis infects the foetus in the womb the baby may be born with swollen arthritic joints. The child might get arthritis when he or she is about 10 years old, especially in the knees and elbows. The knees and elbows are especially affected. Secondary syphilis can lead to symmetrical arthritis of the knees, ankles, shoulders, wrists and the sacroiliac joints at the base of the spine. At this stage of syphilis the arthritis can become chronic.

In tertiary syphilis, the disease has been known to destroy the sensory nerves to the joint and, as there is no sensation of pain, the joint can become damaged without you even realising it. This process especially affects the ankle joint forming a gross, permanent deformity or Charcot's joint. To kill the spirochaete and stop further damage by syphilis you need to take antibiotics during all stages, but your arthritis will only improve at the second stage.

MYCOBACTERIAL ARTHRITIS

Mycobacterium tuberculosis is the bacterium responsible for tuberculosis. It can also induce arthritis in about 1 per cent of people with tuberculosis. Typically, only a single joint is affected at a time, usually the knees, hips or ankles, and progressive pain and swelling of the joint continues over several years. Active lung disease is not common at the time of the arthritis. Diagnosis of tuberculosis-induced arthritis is often hard as the microorganism is difficult to culture, and needs special laboratory stains and culture mediums. Your doctor will probably take a biopsy of joint tissue and then culture it. This is the most sensitive method and will be positive in 90 per cent of cases—taking a sample of joint fluid culture, on the other hand, is only positive in 50 per cent of people.

The incidence of tuberculosis is increasing worldwide and is directly related to the incidence of HIV/AIDS. The immunosuppression of HIV increases the risk of contracting tuberculosis and now doctors will test tuberculosis patients for HIV in order to exclude it. The treatment of tuberculosis-induced arthritis is the same as for lung tuberculosis and involves multiple different antibiotics over six to 12 months. Tuberculosis infections are becoming drug-resistant, and newer antibiotics need to be developed.

TREATMENT FOR TUBERCULOSIS-INDUCED ARTHRITIS IS THE SAME AS FOR LUNG TUBERCULOSIS AND INVOLVES MULTIPLE DIFFERENT ANTIBIOTICS.

Other mycobacteria
Other tuberculosis-related bacterium which also induce arthritis are in the soil—you can pick them up when working in the garden, farming or swimming. Infections of the joint from these bacteria are much less common than infections caused by the tuberculosis bacterium.

FUNGAL ARTHRITIS
Fungal arthritis is very uncommon and is usually spread into the joint via blood from another infected site within the body. Two common fungi to cause arthritis this way are *Coccidiodes immitis* and *Blastomyces dermatitidis*. Direct entry into a joint from trauma (rather than via the blood) may introduce a condition called *Sporothrix schenckii*, which occurs in gardeners who come into contact with sphagnum moss. Men are six times more prone to this than women and people with immune deficiencies or who are alcoholics are also at an increased risk. Nevertheless, don't be afraid to go into the garden for fear of contracting arthritis from this bug. This is a very rare form of arthritis and need not prevent you from enjoying gardening.

Candida albicans (or thrush) can infect a joint, usually the knee, hip or shoulder and especially the spines of intravenous drug users. Other fungal infections, such as *aspergillus* and *cryptococcus*, can be a problem only if your defences have been weakened. You will be treated by having your joint drained and washed out and then with intravenous anti-fungal agents.

VIRAL ARTHRITIS
Viruses can bring on arthritis either by direct infection of the joint or by starting an immune reaction that attacks the joint. The rubella virus, also known as German measles, can cause arthritis in up to 10 per cent of people who contract it or who have been immunised for it. Men are especially susceptible to arthritis from the *mumps* virus. *Parvovirus B19*

is also aggressive in bringing on arthritis—10 per cent of children and 60 per cent of women infected with this virus get arthritis as a complication. Hepatitis B can give a rheumatoid-like condition that's related to the jaundice (yellowing of the skin due to a build-up of bile salts in the body) of this disease. It goes away when the jaundice settles down.

Mosquito-borne viruses, such as Ross River virus, Barmah forest virus, *chikungunya* virus and *O'nyong-nyong* virus can also induce arthritis. HIV is also known to lead to an arthritis similar to Reiter's syndrome (see Chapter 12); if you have psoriasis at the same time, the psoriatic arthritis can flare up.

CHILDHOOD DISEASES SUCH AS GERMAN MEASLES AND MUMPS CAN BE RESPONSIBLE FOR ARTHRITIS.

PARASITIC ARTHRITIS

Infections of joints by parasites are also relatively uncommon, even though some of the parasites are found everywhere. *Giardia intestinalis* and *cryptosporidium* are common parasites found in water and infection with one of them leads to diarrhoea and other bowel infections. Occasionally they can bring on a reactive arthritis. The worms, *strongyloides* and hookworm, also bring on a reactive arthritis. Third world parasites can directly infect joints—the guinea worm, *Dracunculus medinensis*, is responsible for destructive arthritis in the feet, knees and hips as it migrates throughout the body. Another worm, *Wuchereria bancrofti,* can cause filariasis (sometimes called elephantiasis). This leads to an infection in the joint and children are particularly prone to it. Fortunately, this is rare.

CHAPTER | 15

CANARIES AND HEN'S TEETH

W hen I was at medical school, we had a couple of sayings about diseases we didn't expect to encounter in the normal course of events. One is 'canary' for a very rare condition, something you are as likely to see as a canary in a jungle. The other is 'hen's teeth', as canary diseases are as rare as hen's teeth. There are a few unusual types of arthritis that could qualify for a canary or hen's teeth diagnosis.

MIXED CONNECTIVE TISSUE DISEASE

Mixed connective tissue disease is a strange combination of scleroderma, rheumatoid arthritis, systemic lupus erythematosus and polymyositis with its own genetic basis highlighted by an antibody in the blood, anti-U1 RNP. It occurs in all races and usually presents in the 20- to 30-year-old age group and affects more women than men.

MIXED CONNECTIVE TISSUE DISEASE IS A COMBINATION
OF SCLERODERMA, RHEUMATOID ARTHRITIS, LUPUS
AND POLYMYOSITIS. MOST SUFFERERS WILL EVENTUALLY
DEVELOP ONE OF THESE DISEASES AS WELL.

The presenting features of mixed connective tissue disease are Raynaud's phenomenon (see Chapter 9), arthritis, muscle aches, fatigue and, less frequently, fevers, nerve pain and irritation of the lining of the brain. These features may develop over months to years. Sclerodermal changes of the skin are usually restricted to the fingers and toes but occasionally affect the face. Malar butterfly rashes across the face and the discoid-shaped rashes of lupus also occur.

The arthritis of mixed connective tissue disease is similar to that of rheumatoid arthritis and often affects the fingers, hands, wrists and feet. The joint deformities are also similar to those of rheumatoid arthritis. While the lungs also become affected in most people with mixed connective tissue disease, this is not as destructive as it is in scleroderma. Kidney and oesophagus involvement occurs in about one quarter of people, but once again not usually as severely as in scleroderma and lupus. Heart involvement is common with cardiomyopathy (inflammation of the heart muscle) and pericarditis (inflammation of the sac around the heart) occurring. There may also be heart valve problems.

The majority of people with mixed connective tissue disease will eventually develop one of the diseases that make up mixed connective tissue disease—lupus, rheumatoid arthritis, scleroderma or polymyositis. The treatment is essentially the same as for the predominant features of the disease with preservation of essential organ function the overriding goal. The 10-year survival rate for mixed connective tissue disease is approximately 80 per cent, but there are variations depending on which condition finally develops.

DERMATOMYOSITIS OR POLYMYOSITIS

Dermatomyositis and polymyositis are inflammatory diseases that affect muscles (which are anatomically close to joints). Almost one third of people who get these conditions will develop an inflammatory arthritis and sometimes a malignant cancer (up to 10 per cent). Polymyositis means 'many (poly) muscle (myos) inflammation'. Dermatomyositis (skin/muscle/inflammation) also inflames many muscles, as well as the skin, leaving a particular skin rash. The incidence of these diseases is extremely low and affects about five people per million per year—about 90 cases in Australia per year.

Causes and features of dermatomyositis and polymyositis

The cause is unknown, but once again there seems to be an interplay between genetic susceptibility and environmental factors, including infections. Viral infections seem to be the main suspect with similar short-term myositis occurring with *influenzae* virus and *coxsackie* virus infections.

About one third of polymyositis is considered to be primary, which means it's not related to any other disease. You can get it at any age and it's usually slow to progress over months to years. It affects females twice as often as males. The first noticeable symptoms are muscle weakness in the hips, thighs and shoulders making squatting, lifting and climbing stairs difficult, although there is rarely pain associated with the muscle weakness. Other muscles in the body are often spared, but the muscles used for swallowing and the muscles of the gullet may be affected, giving the sensation of food being blocked in the gullet. The heart muscle also can become inflamed, giving you abnormal heart rhythms and heart failure (about 30 per cent of cases). Lung inflammation has also been known.

In dermatomyositis your skin can change either before or after you get muscle symptoms. The skin becomes reddish purple and raised in small patches or more widespread across the body. It may even look like scaly eczema. Usually it develops into a lilac coloured rash that runs across the bridge of the nose, around the eyelids and across the cheeks and which may become itchy. You may also get fluid accumulating around your eyes. Sometimes vasculitis is severe and can block off blood supply to the tissue, resulting in tissue death. The kidney is especially vulnerable. Dermatomyositis affects children in about 20 per cent of cases, but children generally have a better outlook than adult sufferers.

Cancer, especially lung, ovary, breast, colon and lymphoma, is associated with about 10 per cent of cases of dermatomyositis and polymyositis, although this is uncommon in children. The incidence increases with age, especially for those over the age of 60 years. The malignancy may occur up to two years before the occurrence of myositis. In such cases the myositis is secondary to the cancer.

Your doctor will confirm the diagnosis of myositis by elevations of creatinine kinase, a muscle enzyme released into the blood when the muscle cell is damaged, or by electromyograph studies which show altered muscle electrical currents, or by muscle biopsy.

Treatment of dermatomyositis and polymyositis

Cortisone is the treatment, usually given in high doses. Once the condition has stabilised, you can be progressively weaned off the drug. Generally you'll be on cortisone for several years. You can use disease-modifying drugs if you have little response to cortisone or if it helps you come off cortisone quicker. The drugs that may work are azathioprine, methotrexate, cyclosporin and cyclophosphamide.

IF YOU HAVE DERMATOMYOSITIS OR POLYMYOSITIS, IT'S LIKELY THAT YOU'LL NEED LONG-TERM CORTISONE TREATMENT.

The outlook if you have myositis is generally favourable but the mortality rate is about four times greater than for the normal population. The five-year survival rate is about 75 per cent and death is usually associated with kidney, lung or cardiac complications. Women usually have more severe initial problems, and a worse outlook, especially if the myositis is associated with cancer. Most people improve with treatment and usually achieve near normal functioning, although relapses do occur. About 20 per cent of people with the disease need long-term treatment.

BEHCET'S SYNDROME

An extremely rare syndrome, Behcet's is a multi-organ disease that gives recurring oral and genital ulcers, inflammation of the eye, arthritis, brain complications and thrombosis. It affects mostly young adults and the outlook is poorer for men. It's thought to be due to an immune dysfunction because the lesions that induce the problem inflame the blood vessels.

The mouth and genital ulcers have a yellow base and are painful. Occurring either singularly or in clusters, they clear up spontaneously, usually within two weeks, and don't leave a scar. The arthritis associated with Behcet's syndrome usually affects the knees and ankles but doesn't result in any joint destruction. You need quick treatment for eye inflammations, as they can result in blindness. About one quarter of people with Behcet's syndrome develop vein thrombosis or clots, but the risk of forming potentially lethal complications of emboli with clots breaking off and going to the heart and lungs is small. You need to take anti-coagulation medications for this problem.

You can also get thrombosis in the arteries, blocking blood supply to tissues and leading to the death of the organ if a major vessel is affected. Anti-coagulation is also necessary for this complication. You may get pressure around the brain, resulting in psychiatric disturbances and a multiple sclerosis-like syndrome but this is rare.

YOU CAN GET THROMBOSIS (CLOTS) IN BEHCET'S SYNDROME—IF THIS HAPPENS, YOUR DOCTOR WILL PRESCRIBE AN ANTI-COAGULANT. DANGEROUS CLOTS ARE RARE.

Treatment of Behcet's syndrome
Your doctor will usually give you cortisone pastes for the mouth and genital ulcers, colchinine for the arthritis, anti-coagulation for the thrombosis and, if the eyes and brain are affected, oral cortisone and a disease-modifying drug such as azathioprine and cyclosporin.

WHIPPLE'S DISEASE
Whipple's disease is caused by another microbacterium, *Tropheryma whippelii*, which is so small it can only be seen under an electron microscope as it is 0.3 x 1.5 x 2.5 millionths of a metre in size.

Mostly affecting Caucasian men, symptoms include a spectrum of arthritis, prolonged diarrhoea, weight loss, gut malabsorption, fevers, enlarged lymph nodes, inflammation of the heart with heart failure, inflammation of the linings of the heart and lungs, pneumonia, increased skin pigmentation, anaemia, eye inflammation and brain dysfunction, which includes memory loss, blurred vision and confusion. Your doctor will make the diagnosis with a biopsy of the intestine where the lining is virtually replaced by granules that stain magenta with a special PAS stain. The magenta staining has also been shown in the synovium of joints. Electron microscopy will show the presence of the Whipple's bug.

Ninety percent of people who develop Whipple's disease will develop arthritis. The most common joints to be affected are the knees and ankles, although it doesn't last long and rarely permanently damages the joint. The sacroiliac joint between the spine and pelvis does, however, often show damage on X-ray.

JOINTS COMMONLY AFFECTED BY WHIPPLE'S DISEASE ARE THE KNEES AND ANKLES. THERE IS USUALLY NO PERMANENT DAMAGE TO THESE JOINTS.

Treatment of Whipple's disease

Whipple's disease is now curable with antibiotics—usually a combination antibiotic of trimethoprim and sulfamethoxazole which has to be taken for at least 12 months. Other antibiotics have been used but relapse rates are high, while trimethoprim with sulfamethoxazole can bring on remission and even lead to complete disappearance of the magenta-staining granules.

INFLAMMATORY BOWEL DISEASE

Ther two main causes of inflammatory bowel disease are Crohn's disease and ulcerative colitis—about 20 per cent of people with one of these diseases will develop a form of arthritis.

If the large bowel is inflamed, or there are complications of haemorrhage, abscess formation or eye inflammation, you will have a higher chance of developing arthritis, which will usually come on suddenly and be associated with bowel flare ups. The arthritis usually only lasts six months and doesn't permanently damage the joint. The ankles, knees and hips are the joints most usually inflamed, although the inflammation may migrate around the body between joints. The arthritis responds to the treatment of the bowel disease with cortisone, sulfasalazine and methotrexate. It's best to avoid non-steroidal anti-inflammatories because of their effect on the gut and the risk of ulceration, perforation and haemorrhage. Cox-2 inhibitors should be safe.

Inflammatory bowel disease also has an association with ankylosing spondylitis (see Chapter 12)—up to 43 per cent of people with inflammatory bowel disease will develop a form of spinal inflammation. The converse is also true—5 per cent of people with ankylosing spondylitis will develop inflammatory bowel disease. Men are more likely to develop spinal inflammation that is unrelated to the activity of their bowel disease. Typical symptoms are back pain and stiffness after rest, although the symptoms are somewhat relieved with exercise. An eye inflammation is also common with the spinal inflammation. X-rays usually confirm arthritis of the sacroiliac joint and treatment is the same as for ankylosing spondylitis. Unfortunately ankylosing spondilitis doesn't spontaneously resolve itself like other arthritis associated with inflammatory bowel disease.

ACROMEGALY

The pituitary gland lies at the base of the brain—one of its specialised functions is to produce growth hormone. If there's a benign tumour of the cells that produce growth hormone, too much will be produced and acromegaly (or gigantism) will be the result.

Acromegaly is a chronic disease associated with bony and soft tissue overgrowth, resulting in increased sizes of the hand, foot, head, jaw, tongue and any other tissue dependent on growth hormone. It can affect eyesight, block the sinuses, give a deepening of the voice, entrap nerves, especially at the wrist giving carpal tunnel syndrome, cause diabetes and high blood pressure with heart failure and sleep apnoea.

In joints, there's bony and cartilage overgrowth leading to destructive osteoarthritis. Knees, shoulders, hips and hands are often affected. The new cartilage that's produced in acromegaly is faulty and easily fissures, ulcerates and breaks down. Ligaments become overgrown due to excess growth hormone and lose their strength becoming lax. Abnormal forces then act on the joint leading to further cartilage destruction. Secondary gout and pseudogout may also develop in the joint. Ligament laxity in the lower spine will bring on back pain and after several years this may progress to osteoarthritis. You may also develop Raynaud's phenomenon (see Chapter 9).

Treatment of acromegaly

Acromegaly can be held in check by removal of the tumour from the pituitary, either by surgery or by radiation therapy. If the tumour is fully removed, a lot of the soft tissue overgrowth will recede but any bony overgrowth remains. If you've developed osteoarthritis, this is permanent and needs to be treated the same way as normal osteoarthritis (see Chapter 5).

HAEMOCHROMATOSIS

Haemochromatosis is a disease where too much iron is absorbed from the gut and is then deposited in tissues within the body where it shouldn't be. The tissue becomes damaged and you can get organ failure. This is an inherited disease and appears to be of Celtic/European origin—one in 10 in these populations are carriers, although only 0.3 per cent of the population actually has the disorder. Men are affected up to 10 times more than women. It takes some time for the iron overload to happen and damage the tissue, so you won't notice symptoms straight away and if you're under 20 you probably won't have symptoms. But once the tissues are damaged there are serious consequences. The heart can develop cardiomyopathy and abnormal heart rhythms, the liver becomes cirrhotic and may develop cancers, the skin takes on a bronzed pigmentation and the pancreas is damaged, leading to diabetes.

WHEN TISSUES ARE DAMAGED AS A RESULT OF HAEMOCHROMATOSIS, THERE ARE INCREASED RISKS FOR THE HEART, THE LIVER AND THE PANCREAS.

About 40 per cent of people with haemochromatosis develop arthritis, usually after the age of 50 years. The arthritis looks like osteoarthritis with an inflammatory component and often first affects the small joints of the hands, followed by the larger joints of the body. Secondary CPPD pseudogout may also form in the haemochromatosis-affected joints. A biopsy of the joint synovium can show the iron within both the synovial and cartilage cells.

IRON DAMAGES THE JOINT CARTILAGE BY INDUCING THE PRODUCTION OF SUPEROXIDES WITHIN THE CARTILAGE AND BREAKING IT DOWN, THEREBY INTERFERING WITH COLLAGEN FORMATION.

Treatment of haemochromatosis

Treatment for the arthritis of haemochromatosis is limited to non-steroidal anti-inflammatory medications and analgesics. Treatment of the iron overload is by regular blood letting to decrease the total iron amount in the body, but this doesn't improve the arthritis.

HAEMOPHILIA AND ARTHRITIS

Haemophilia is a genetic disorder that leads to a lack of production of a blood protein, factor VIII, that allows blood to clot. With little or no factor VIII the body can't stop itself bleeding, leading to haemorrhage. Spontaneous bleeding into joint cavities is common—the degree of bleeding depends on the degree of haemophilia. Bleeding into joints becomes evident early in life—you'll often notice it in the early toddler years when your child has learned to stand and walk, frequently falling in the process, and getting a haemarthrosis (blood in the joint). The joint becomes hot and swollen and, because the blood is unable to clot, it remains in liquid form within the joint. Over a period of a week or so, the blood is reabsorbed out of the joint back into the body and the joint returns somewhat back to normal.

Recurrent bleeds into a joint eventually lead to chronic arthritis, and the affected joint can become permanently deformed. If there is bleeding into a muscle, the muscle can become internally deranged and exert abnormal forces on the joint. This in itself also can lead to chronic arthritis and permanently damaged joints. The chronic arthritis of haemophilia is similar to osteoarthritis.

IN HAEMOPHILIA, RECURRENT BLEEDS INTO A JOINT EVENTUALLY RESULT IN CHRONIC ARTHRITIS OF THAT JOINT.

Another complication of haemophilia is the increased risk of infective arthritis, which may make it difficult to differentiate from a bleed from the haemophilia. If your doctor suspects an infection, he or she will drain the joint immediately and give you intravenous antibiotics.

Treatment of haemophilia

Your doctor will treat haemarthrosis by giving factor VIII intravenously at the first sign of haemorrhage. Analgesics are safe to use and short-term use of non-steroidal anti-inflammatory medications is considered safe and effective in relieving symptoms. Avoid long-term use because of the risk of haemorrhage from peptic ulcers. The bleeding tendencies of non-steroidals are not an issue with haemophiliacs as they don't affect the clotting factors, but a cox-2 inhibitor would be considered safer. In severe cases of chronic arthritis in haemophilia, you may need to have overgrowths of synovium excised, radioactive destruction of the synovium with yttrium 90, or total joint replacement. Any surgery you consider must be done with intravenous factor VIII replacement during and after surgery.

SICKLE CELL DISEASE

Sickle cell disease is a genetic disease of red blood cells in which the protein that carries oxygen to the rest of the body—haemoglobin—has an abnormal structure that leads to stiffening and distortion of the red blood cell, giving a curved or sickle shape to the cell, or 'sickling' of the red blood cell. The result is the inability of the red blood cell to cross the very small blood vessels (capillaries), so the tissues aren't supplied with oxygen. The red blood cells can alternate between the normal shape and the sickled state. When they change to the sickled state you will develop symptoms as the blood doesn't transfer oxygen very efficiently. This is termed a 'sickle crisis'.

The specific damage done to joints if you have sickle cell disease results from the loss of blood supply. The joint becomes inflamed and swollen and surrounding soft tissues also become inflamed. The synovium, cartilage, bone and bone marrow of the joint die off and you experience intense pain. If the ball of the femur in the hip joint is affected in this way (avascular necrosis), secondary osteoarthritis develops and you'll eventually need a hip replacement. Other joints are affected in a similar way. People with sickle cell disease are at an increased risk of infective arthritis involving different joints. There is also an increased risk of gouty arthritis due to the increased turnover of red blood cells in sickle cell disease resulting in increased urate production.

IF YOU HAVE SICKLE CELL DISEASE, YOU HAVE A HIGHER RISK OF GETTING INFECTIVE ARTHRITIS AND GOUT.

Treatment of sickle cell disease

There is no cure for sickle cell disease as it's a genetically based disease. You will need to avoid anything that might bring on a sickling crisis such as other infections, dehydration, excessive exercise, anxiety or abrupt changes in temperature. Treatment will give you symptom relief only.

THALASSAEMIA

Thalassaemia is another genetic defect of the haemoglobin protein that carries oxygen in the red blood cells around the body. Haemoglobin is composed of several chains of proteins and if there is a defect in production of one of those chains anaemia can develop. Associated with this is a defect in the bone structure resulting in the arthritis of thalassaemia. Any joint can be affected, but it seems that the ankles are the most common site. The severity and chronicity of arthritis is highly variable. Basically calcium is lost from the bone of the joint, resulting in the development of microfractures of the bone. The synovium swells up and damages the cartilage. It's thought the abnormal iron metabolism associated with thalassaemia damages the joint structures although this is not well understood. Gouty arthritis and infective arthritis are also an increased risk with thalassaemia.

Treatment of thalassaemia

Thalassaemia has no cure—you'll need to have iron levels monitored and control excess iron levels within the blood. Arthritis treatment is again restricted to symptom relief as for sickle cell disease.

GLOSSARY

adrenal glands: glands located directly above the kidneys that release cortisol, aldosterone (a fluid/electrolyte-controlling hormone) and adrenaline-type hormones into the blood.

amino acids: a group of organic molecules of nitrogen, carbon, oxygen and hydrogen used as the building blocks for different proteins within the body.

anaemia: a low number of red blood cells leading to a low oxygen-carrying capacity in the blood, giving symptoms of tiredness, lethargy and shortness of breath.

antibodies: see immunoglobulins.

arthritis: inflammation of a joint.

arthroscopy: insertion of a telescope-like instrument into the joint cavity. Used to assess the joint for damage to the cartilage, bone and ligaments.

articular: of the joints.

bacteria: microscopic single cell organisms that are able to invade other organisms or release chemicals that destroy other cells on which they feed.

bone marrow: the soft tissue inside a bone that produces the different cells that constitute the blood.

bradykinin: a protein whose function is to swell the blood vessels and surrounding tissue when these are inflamed.

chondrocytes: cells that produce cartilage.

cirrhosis: liver cells are destroyed and replaced by non-functioning fibrotic scar tissue.

collagen: the protein produced by bone cells, cartilage cells and fibroblasts in the skin, which acts to hold the cells of an organ together.

connective tissue: the tissue throughout the body that holds the cells of each organ together.

contracture: the joint is fixed in a position and cannot move through its full range of movement.

cortisol: a naturally occurring steroid produced by the adrenal glands. Involved in the control of glucose levels in the blood, bone control, inflammation and immune function.

cortisone: a synthetically produced steroid, chemically related to cortisol that performs the same functions within the body.

cyclo-oxgenase: also known as COX, an enzyme found in the body involved in prostaglandin production.

deep vein thrombosis: the blood solidifies or clots within a deep-sited vein in the body. Can lead to a pulmonary embolus which is life-threatening.

DNA: deoxyribonucleic acid. Large-weight proteins in the nucleus of cells that form into double helical strands and form the genetic material of cells.

electrolyte levels: the levels of salts in the blood and cells of the body. Includes sodium, potassium, chloride and calcium.

enzyme: proteins produced by cells to speed up the chemical reactions in the body.

extra-articular: away from the joint. Applies to bodily effects of a disease that do not involve the joint.

fibroblasts: skin cells that make collagen and connective tissue for the skin.

fungi: a lower form of plant life that can cause disease inside the human body.

gastrointestinal system: consists of the oesophagus, stomach, small and large intestines, liver and pancreas.

glucose: a naturally occurring sugar that is the main chemical used by the human body to produce energy needs.

haemarthrosis: blood within the joint cavity.

hepatitis: inflammation of the liver. Can be due to a viral infection with viruses or an auto-immune disorder.

histamine: an organic molecule of nitrogen, carbon and hydrogen found throughout the body and involved in control of stomach acid secretion, muscle function and blood vessel leakiness in inflammation.

human tumour necrosis factor: a protein, released by macrophages of the immune system, that promotes inflammation and helps kill tumours and germs.

hyperuricaemia: high levels of urate in the blood.

immune system: consists of lymph glands, bone marrow, spleen and liver. Produces the white blood cells that fight infections and repair the body.

immunoglobulins: proteins produced by lymphocytes that are either released into the blood stream or are coated on the lymphocytes' cell wall. They recognise micro-organisms that invade the body resulting in stimulation of the immune system to fight the infection.

interleukins: proteins, produced and released by the immune system's white blood cells, that increase the inflammatory effect and help fight infection.

intra-articular: inside the joint. Injections can be given this way.

intra-muscular: inside the muscles. Injections can be given this way.

intravenous: inside the vein. Injections can be given this way directly into the blood stream.

inflammation: the immune system is stimulated to promote healing. The organ involved shows signs of redness, swelling, heat, pain and loss of function.

interferon: a lymphokine protein of the immune system involved in inflammation and fighting viruses.

leucotrienes: proteins released by neutrophil cells that promote an inflammatory effect.

lymphocytes: a subgroup of white blood cells that recognise and help identify germs within the body by releasing the chemicals immunoglobulins and lymphokines.

lymphokines: a group of proteins of the immune system released by lymphocytes that help macrophages recognise and destroy bacteria.

lysosomes: small packages of enzymes within cells that when released lead to cell and debris breakdown.

macrophage: a large white blood cell found throughout the body in blood and tissues that scavenge dead cells, foreign matter and germs. A type of phagocyte.

metabolism: the chemical reactions that occur within the body to produce its energy requirements.

mucopolysaccharides: another name for proteoglycans. Molecules of sugar and protein.

neutrophils: a subgroup of white blood cells that are highly mobile and engulf germs leading to their destruction by the release of enzymes from lysosomes.

ophthalmologist: a doctor who specialises in diseases of the eye.

osteoblasts: bone cells that produce new bone matrix. Work in equilibrium with osteoclasts to maintain healthy bone tissue.

osteoclasts: bone cells that destroy old and damaged bone.

osteopaenia: loss of calcium in the bone. A mild form of osteoporosis.

osteophytes: the bony spurring that occurs along the rim of an osteoarthritic joint.

osteoporosis: loss of bone where the bone becomes less dense and is at risk of fracturing. Not to be confused with osteoarthritis which is a degenerative arthritis.

pancreatitis: inflammation of the pancreas in the abdomen.

pannus: an overgrowth of the synovial cells of a joint which leads to bone and cartilage destruction in some forms of inflammatory arthritis.

parathyroid glands: a series of small glands in the neck which control calcium levels within the body and bones.

pericarditis: inflammation of the sac around the heart.

phagocytes: cells of the immune system which are the scavengers, ingesting and destroying germs and debris. Includes the neutrophils and macrophages.

photosensitive: a reaction to ultraviolet light or sunlight.

pituitary gland: a small gland that hangs off the underside of the brain. It releases hormones that control the thyroid gland, growth patterns of the body, electrolyte mechanisms and sexual organs of the body.

placebo: a 'medication' without any pharmacological effect.

polymorphonuclear leucocytes: see neutrophils.

polymyositis: an inflammatory condition that strikes many muscles of the body (poly = many, myo = muscle, it is = inflammation).

prostaglandins: molecules of carbon and fatty acids that occur throughout the body involved in controlling the nervous system, reproduction, circulation and immune system functions.

proteins: nitrogen-based molecules within the body composed of series of amino acids that have multitudinous functions inside and outside cells.

proteoglycans: a larger molecule containing building blocks of proteins and sugars.

rheumatologist: a doctor who has done post-graduate training in internal medicine and diseases of the musculoskeletal system, especially the joints.

rhinitis: inflammation of the nasal passages giving sneezing and an itchy, runny nose.

RNA: ribonucleic acid. Large-weight molecules found in cells that act as transport messenger proteins in cell function.

septic: the toxic effect when the body is infected by a micro-oganism.

synovium or synovial membrane: a joint tissue consisting of a thin layer of synovial cells that produce the lubricating fluid of joints. Found lining a joint cavity, tendon sheaths or bursae.

thrombosis: the formation of a clot within a blood vessel.

tinnitus: hearing abnormal ringing or other noises that aren't present, caused by a malfunction of the hearing system.

uveitis: an inflammation of the uvea, the pigmented layer of the iris of the eye.

vasculitis: inflammation of the blood vessels.

virus: a structure comprised of a protein coat with either DNA or RNA inside. Able to infect other living organisms and needs to do so to be able to reproduce. Ranges in size from 10 to 250 nanometres.

APPENDIX I
DRUG NAMES

A particular drug may have several names—initially there is an experimental name, such as XP-23, while the drug is still being researched, then a pharmaceutical name, such as celecoxib, and then a brand name, such as Celebrex. If the drug is then marketed by more than one pharmaceutical company there will be several brand names for the same drug from each company. Pharmaceutical companies also sometimes use different brand names in different countries because they claim different names have different connotations.

Each drug is listed below by pharmaceutical name; it is then followed by several brand names for that drug.

SIMPLE ANALGESICS
paracetamol: Panadol, Panamax, Dymadon, Tylenol, Herron, Febridol, Setamol, Tempra.

NARCOTIC ANALGESICS
codeine: Codalgin, Panadeine forte, Codral forte, Dymadon forte, Codeine phosphate, Mersyndol forte, Prodeine.

dextropropoxyphene: Digesic, Capadex, Paradex, Doloxene.

oxycodone: Endone.

morphine: Morphine sulphate, Morphine tartrate, Mnamorph, Kapanol, MS Contin, Morphalgin, Ordine.

NON-STEROIDAL ANTI-INFLAMMATORIES
salicylic acid: Aspirin, Aspro, Alka-seltzer, Bex, Disprin, Ecotrin, Solprin, Spren, Vincents powders.

naproxen: Naprosyn, Anaprox, Inza, Proxen sr.

ibuprofen: Act-3, Actiprofen, Brufen, Nurofen, Rafen.

ketoprofen: Oruvail, Orudis.

diclofenac: Fenac, Voltaren, Diclohexal.

indomethacin: Indocid, Hicin, Arthrexin.

piroxicam: Candyl, Feldene, Pirox, Mobilis, Rosig.

sulindac: Saldac, Clinoril, Aclin.

diflunisal: Dolobid.

mefanamic acid: Mefic, Ponstan.

tiaprofenic acid: Surgam.

tenoxicam: Tilcotil.

ketorolac: Toradol.

COX-2 INHIBITORS
celecoxib: Celebrex.

rofecoxib: Vioxx.

NATUROPATHIC MEDICATIONS
glucosamine: Arthro-total, OsteoEze, Arthro-aid, Osteo-relief, Arthoflex, Bioglan, Golden-glow, Healthstream arthritis relief, Procosamine.

CORTISONE-BASED DRUGS
Prednisolone, Solone, Prednisone, Celestone, Hydroxycortisone, Betametasone, Trimcinolone, Methylprednisolone, Dexamethasone.

DISEASE-MODIFYING DRUGS
sulfasalazine: Salazopyrin, Pyralin.

D-penicillamine: D-penamine.

hydroxychloroquine: Plaquenil.

gold: Auranofin, Sodium aurothiomalate, Sodium aurothioglucose.

methotrexate: Ledertrexate, Methoblastin.

azathioprine: Imuran, Thioprine.

cyclosporin: Neoral, Sandimmun.

cyclophosphamide: Cycloblastin, Endoxan-asta.

leflunomide: Arava.

APPENDIX 2
FURTHER
INFORMATION

Arthritis Foundation of Australia
National Office: 52 Parramatta Rd, Forest Lodge, NSW 2037
Phone: (02) 9552 6085

New South Wales: 13 Harold St, North Parramatta 2151
Phone: (02) 9683 1622 www.arthritisnsw.org.au

Victoria: 263 Kooyong Rd, Elsternwick 3185
Phone: (03) 9530 0255 www.arthritisvic.org.au

Australian Capital Territory: Health Promotion Centre,
Childers St, Canberra City 2600
Phone: (02) 6257 4842

Queensland: 134A St Pauls Terrace, Spring Hill 4000
Phone: (07) 3831 4255 www.arthritis.org.au

South Australia: 1/202 Glen Osmond Rd, Fullarton 5063
Phone: (08) 8379 5711

Western Australia: 17 Lemnos St, Shenton Park 6008
Phone: (08) 9388 2199 www.arthritiswa.org.au

Tasmania: McDougall Building, Ellerslie Rd, Battery Point 7004
Phone: (03) 6234 4689 www.tased.edu.au/tasonline/raft

Northern Territory: Nightcliff Commmunity Centre, 18 Bauhinia St, Nightcliff 0810
Phone: (08) 8948 5232 www.oct4.net.au/afnt

INDEX

Page numbers in *italics* refer to diagrams and tables